The Calendar Cookbook

In deep appreciation I dedicate this book to my father and mother, to my teachers George and Lima Ohsawa and to all our friends.

The Calendar Cookbook

by Cornellia Aihara

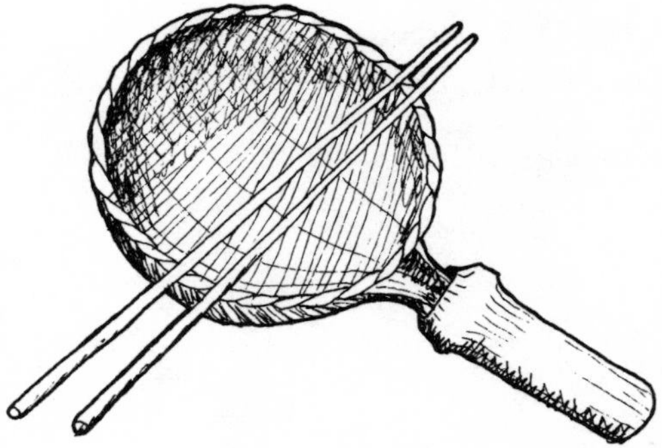

George Ohsawa Macrobiotic Foundation
Oroville, California

Books by the same author:

Chico-San Cookbook
Macrobiotic Child Care
Do of Cooking - 4 volumes
Soybean Diet - with Herman Aihara

These and other related titles available from:

George Ohsawa Macrobiotic Foundation
1544 Oak Street
Oroville, California 95965

ISBN 0-918860-32-6

Acknowledgments

After the French Meadows Summer Camp sponsored by the George Ohsawa Macrobiotic Foundation in 1972, I looked over the menus of the meals I served at camp. In revising them, I had the idea to keep a one-year record of menus. I thought this would be a practical, everyday help for those people beginning to cook.

One year later, I began work with my best friend, Mrs. Hazel Lerman. She worked very hard, transcribing by hand from my broken English. Next, Ms. Joanne Kowalenok and Ms. Alice Feinberg typed the first version.

Since then, seven years passed. G.O.M.F. moved from San Francisco to Oroville. We started Vega Institute and Herman and I both became very busy and could not work on the cookbook. I deeply appreciate two Vega students, Ms. Lisa McKinney and Ms. Sally Chaney, who both helped with typing. After we temporarily discontinued Vega, Ms. Betty Patterson began corrections on the book.

Later, we made the final revisions and typed the manuscript again. Finally, we got our new typesetting machine at the Foundation and we became ready to finish the book. For illustrations I asked Nan Schleiger, who did the work in the *Chico-San Cookbook*; for the cover, Carl Campbell of San Francisco, who did the illustrations in my four-volume *Do of Cooking*.

I am fifty-three years old and have a poor school education but I think this is a good cookbook. Without the help of our many friends I could not have finished this book; I express my gratitude to them because they study the *unique principle* of George Ohsawa. Again I say thank you to volunteers Hazel, Joanne, Betty, Alice, Lisa and Sally. As soon as possible I will enjoy giving them each a copy of the book in my appreciation for their efforts.

My mother often said, "You never finish what you start. You must learn to finish." She tried to teach me knitting but I wouldn't complete my work. Now, I finish my knitting – very fast. And, even though from beginning to end it took seven years, finally I finish this cookbook.

I would like to thank the final production staff: Sandy Rothman, editing; Carl Ferre, design and layout; Lois Engelkes, typesetting.

Cornellia Aihara
Oroville, California
May 15, 1979

From the Author

I wrote this book for those people who are just beginning macrobiotics. For one year I served these dishes at the George Ohsawa Macrobiotic Foundation. You can use this book to discover how to balance food and make new combinations, such as deep-fried foods combined with boiled green vegetables or bean sauce combined with seaweed. There are also many party dishes: New Year's, Christmas, Thanksgiving, 4th of July, wedding menu, children's birthday menu plus summer and autumn camp menus which have recipes for foods cooked outdoors.

These menus were created by considering the weather, season, economy and the individual's condition. In winter I prepared warm dishes for the cold days. On special occasions such as the birthday of one of the children I served a regular American dinner. This was a rare occasion for us to eat this way and I balanced the dinner according to yin and yang.

The most important ingredient for a good cook is love. When you are having a party, think of your guests and their likes and serve them food which they will enjoy. Your party will be a success.

Many people say that macrobiotic cooking takes lots of time. I hope that this book will save you time by giving you menus and an idea of balance. Please find out for yourself how much fun it is to cook. I enjoy cooking very much myself and moreover I enjoy the feeling from the people eating my food — their relaxed and smiling faces, happy conversation and gratitude for a good dinner. Please make yourself a good and beautiful cook with your love. From this your family and friends will become healthy and happy.

For this reason I wrote this new cookbook. I have written other cookbooks, the *Chico-San Cookbook* and *Do of Cooking*; please refer to these books to expand your understanding of macrobiotic cooking and philosophy.

Thank you for reading this cookbook. I hope that we meet somewhere, sometime and that you will be a good cook — one who makes your self, family, friends and the whole world happy.

Cornellia Aihara
San Francisco, California
January 1, 1973

Contents

Foreword

This cookbook may be used in several ways. It may be followed as a daily menu guide through the twelve months of the year – two meals per day. The menu section can be used as a reference for sample meals, seasonal balance or combining leftovers. The topical index may be used to find recipes for a certain dish or type of food. A standard index is also provided.

The menu section contains a daily record of what Cornellia served for each meal during one entire year. She sometimes changes recipes according to season, balance, availability and other conditions; these variations are indicated in the menu section. Similarly, the name of a given recipe can also change to reflect a slight variation. When in doubt, refer to the recipe number.

Days and dates given are for 1973. In other years, days and dates may not coincide. Please make this slight adjustment. The day of the week is more important to Cornellia as she prepares different meals on the weekends. You will also want to celebrate your own festive days; for ideas, refer to the guide to festive meals at the beginning of the menu section. Although not listed, bancha tea was usually served after each meal.

In order to avoid confusion, *all numbers refer to recipe numbers.* No page numbers have been included.

Cutting Styles

Kirikata: How to cut

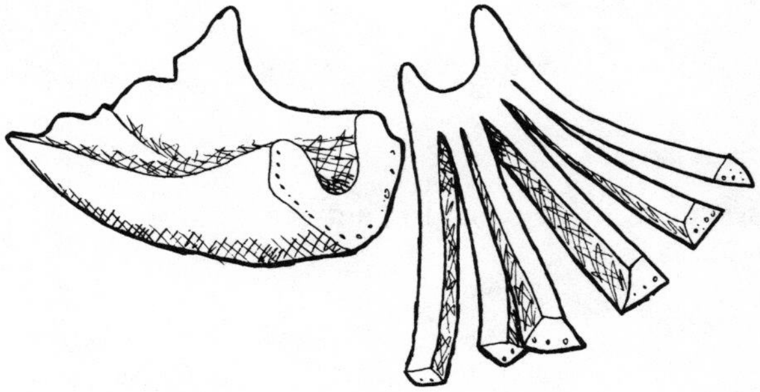

Koguchigiri

Ko means small, *guchi* means end or edge. *Giri* means cut.

Cut thin rounds, straight across the vegetable.

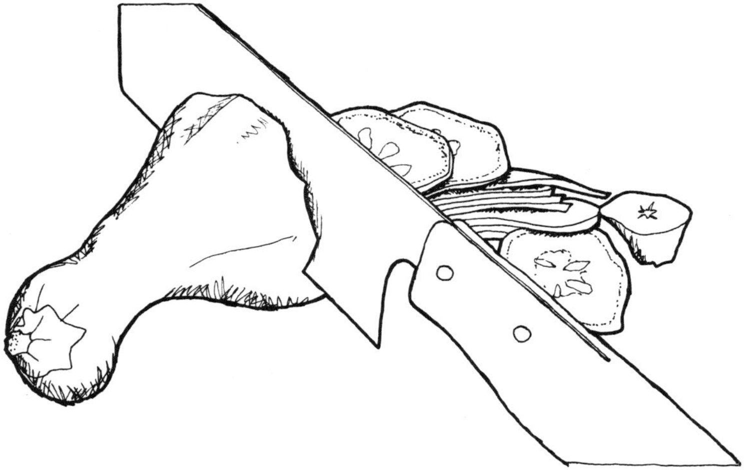

Wagiri

Wa means circle.

This is similar to koguchigiri, but the rounds are cut thicker.

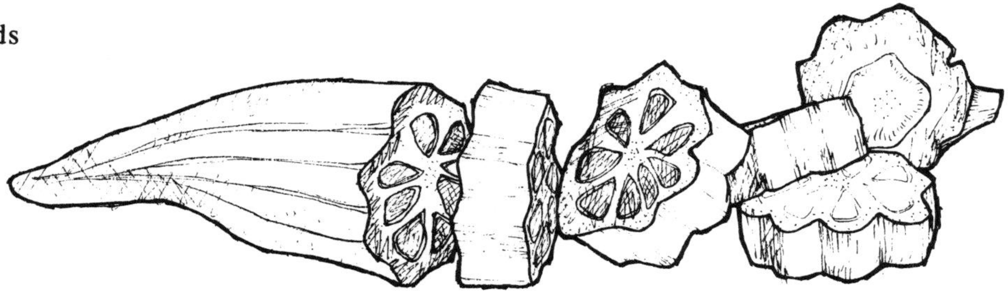

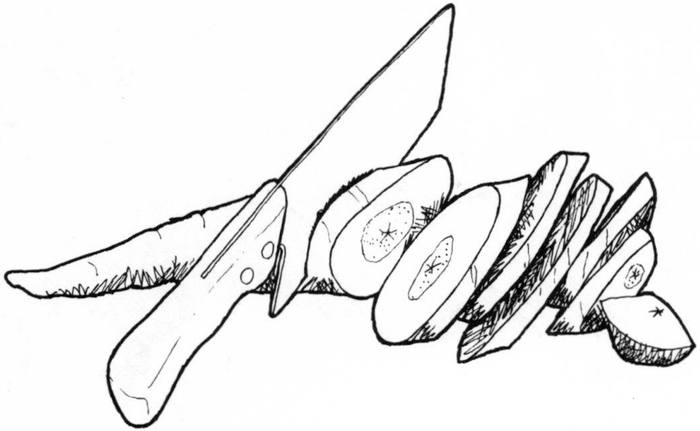

Hasugiri

Hasu means diagonal.

This is a balanced cut. Each piece has part of the yin end and part of the yang end as well as part of the outside and part of the inside of the vegetable.

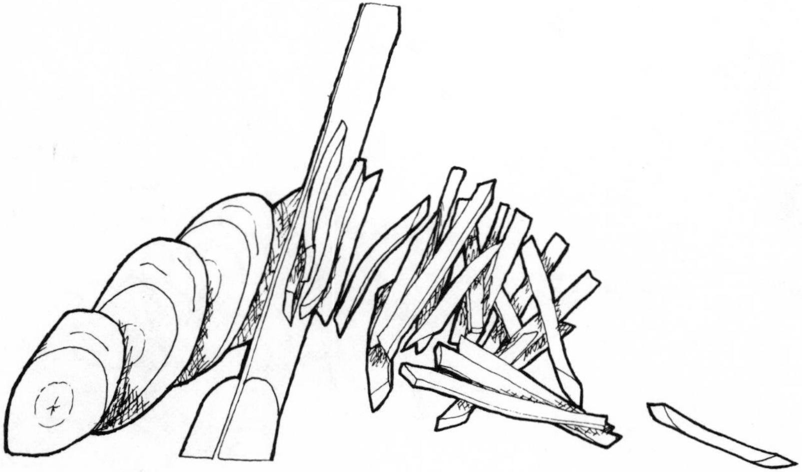

Sengiri

Two words have the sound of *sen* — one means thousand, the other means line. The style of cutting in a thousand lines is known as matchsticks, or julienne.

Hangetsugiri

Han is half, *getsu* is moon.

To cut these half-moons, first cut the vegetable in half lengthwise. Then cut across, koguchigiri style.

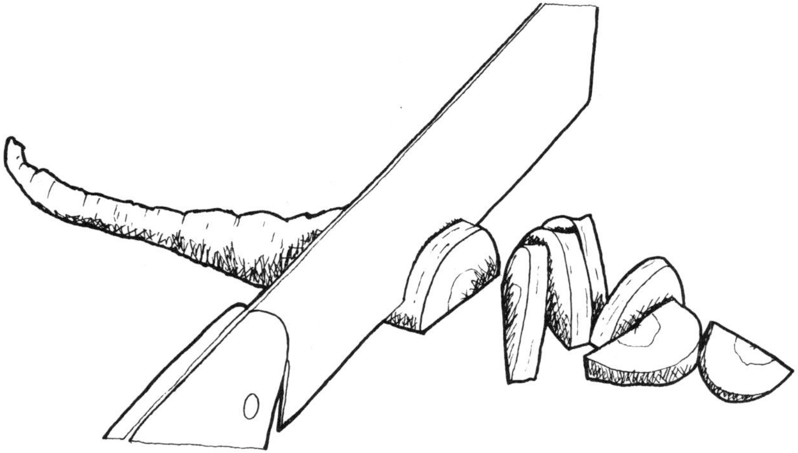

Ichogiri

Icho is the Japanese name for the gingko tree, which has a heart-shaped leaf.

Cut in half lengthwise as in hangetsu, then in half lengthwise again. Then cut across, koguchigiri.

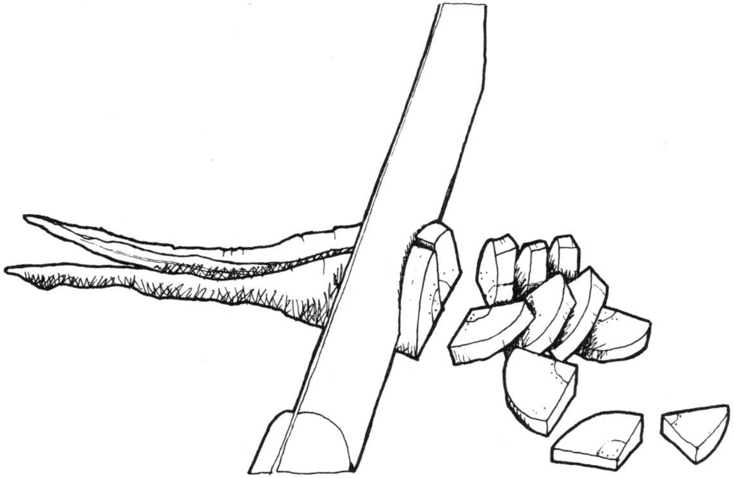

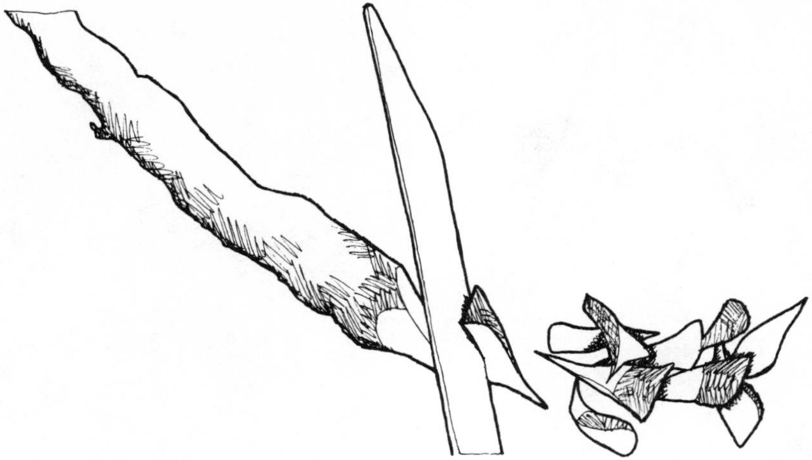

Sasagaki

Sasa is a small bamboo leaf and *gaki* means to shave.

Begin at the pointed end and shave as though sharpening a pencil, rotating the vegetable with each knife cut. The shavings may be as thick or long as desired.

This is a traditional cutting style for burdock but it can be used with carrot, daikon or any long vegetable.

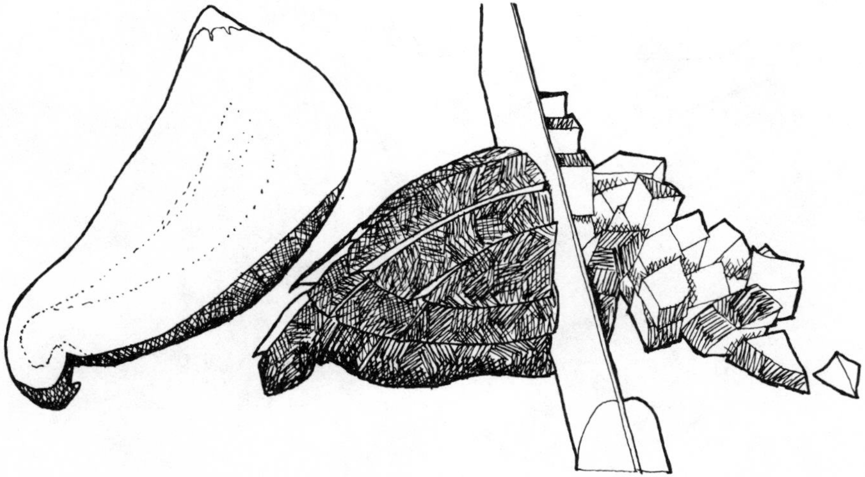

Sainome

Sai is dice (gambling) and *nome* means the face of the dice.

The size of the cubes depends on the recipe and the vegetable.

Mawashigiri

Mawashi means to turn.

Cut vegetable in half vertically, then turn on its axis and cut into half-moon-shaped slices.

This is a balanced way to cut round vegetables — there is part of the root and part of the top in each slice.

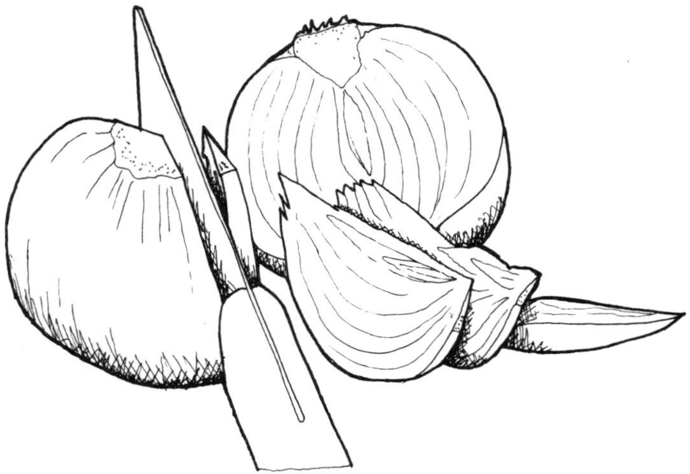

Mijingiri

Mijin means particle of dust.

Finely mince by slicing thinly in opposite directions. Keep attached at root so it will be easier to cut, then chop root.

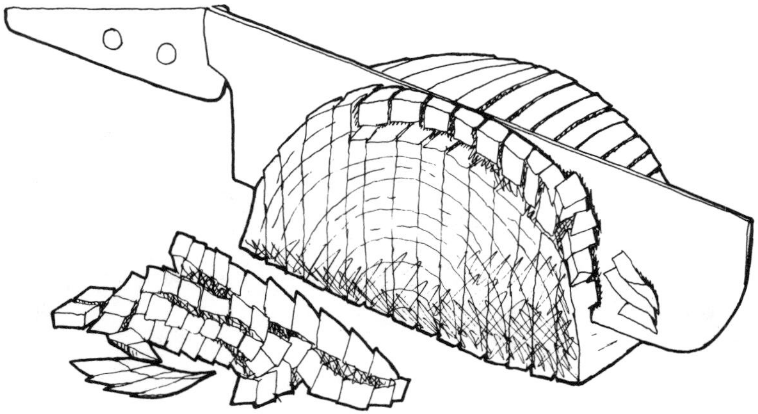

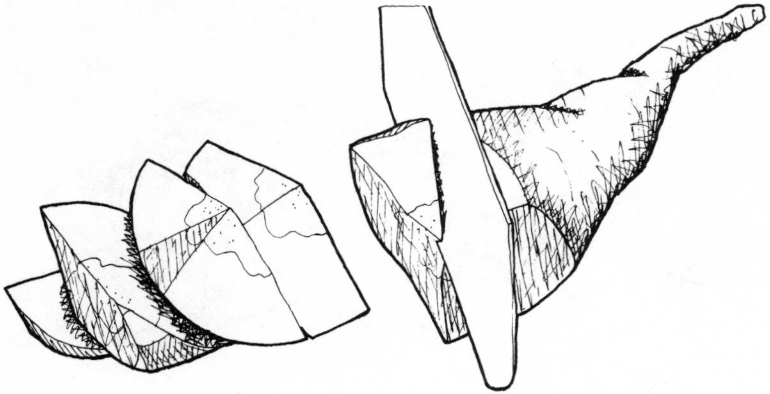

Rangiri

Ran means irregular.

Make a diagonal cut, then turn 180 degrees and make a diagonal cut in the same direction. Continue. These diagonal wedges are large but will cook quickly.

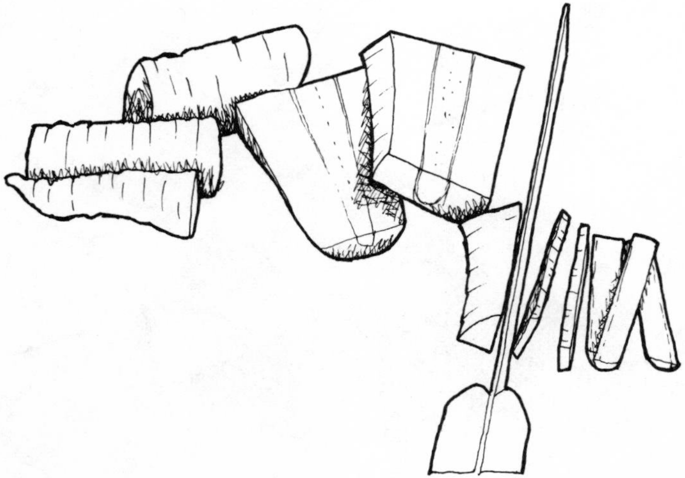

Tanzaku

Tanzaku is the long, thin paper favored by Oriental calligraphers.

Cut vegetable into sections 1½″ long, then slice into vertical pieces. Lay pieces on largest face and slice lengthwise, fairly thin.

Kikukagiri

Kikuka are chrysanthemum flowers.

Make thin cuts in opposite directions. A chopstick on either side of the vegetable keeps it attached at the base.

Soak the cut vegetable (such as radish) in ice water and it will open up like a flower.

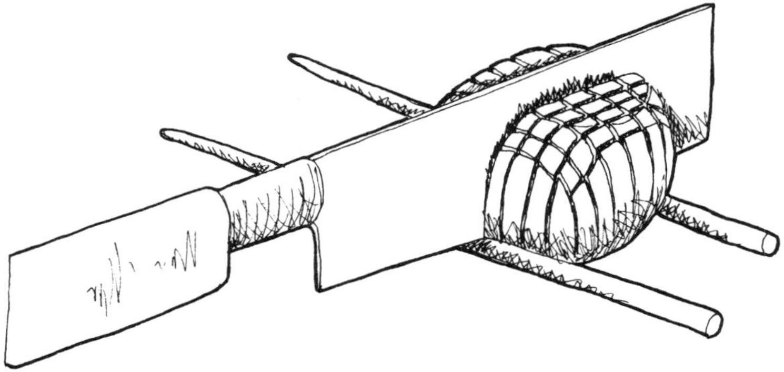

Kikko

Kikko is tortoise shell.

Cut a grille pattern into the vegetable without going all the way through.

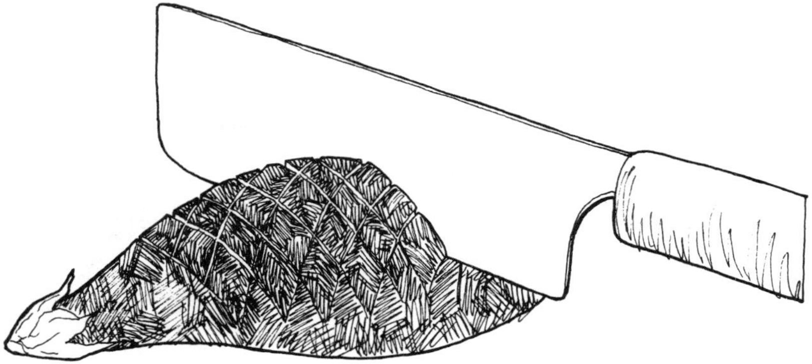

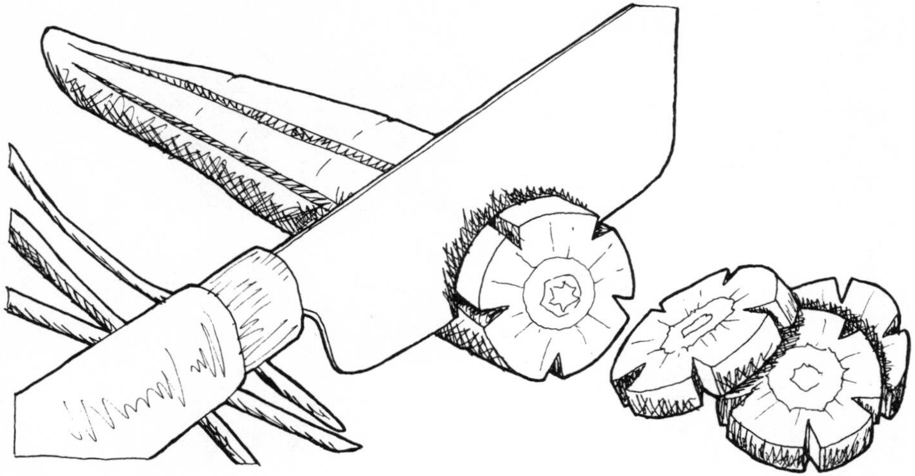

Hanagata

Hana means flower.

Cut small, thin wedges lengthwise 4 or 5 times around the vegetable. Then slice into rounds to make flower shape.

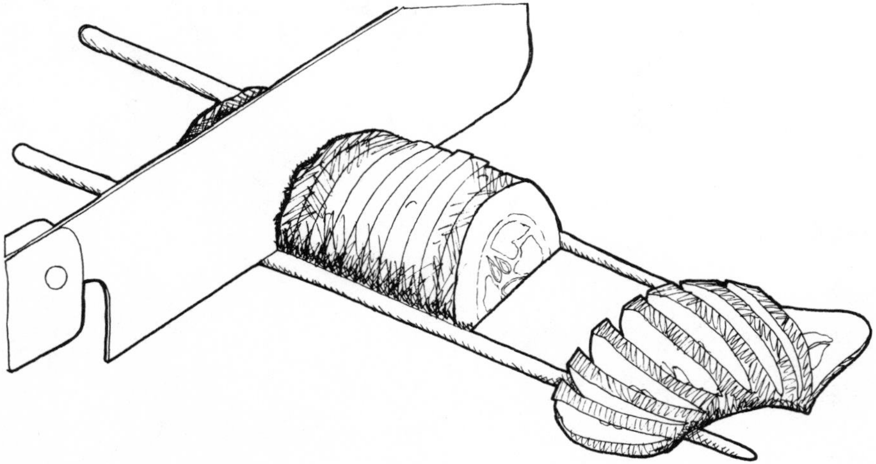

Suehiro

Suehiro means fan-shaped.

Soak in ice water to open. This is a symbol for further development: the hope that the future will open for you.

Topical Index

Grains

Noodles

Vegetables

Sea Vegetables

Fish and Animal

Soups and Potages

Beans

Pickles

Salads

Condiments

Dressings and Sauces

Beverages

Bread and Flour

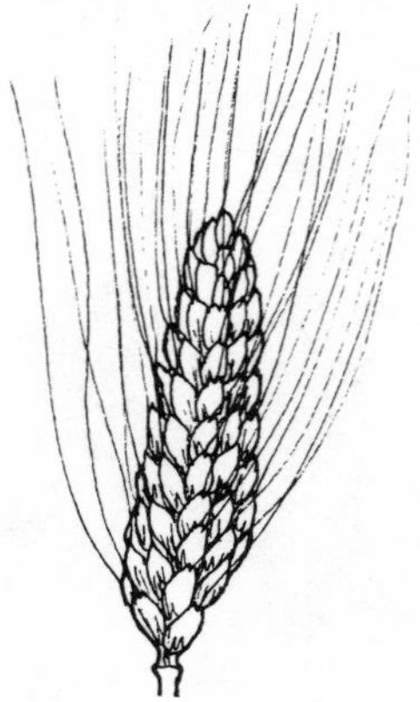

Desserts

Miscellaneous

Recipes

Azuki Bean Rice 1a.

2 cups brown rice
½ cup azuki beans
3½ cups cold water
½ tsp. sea salt

Wash the rice and beans together (see 1b. for washing rice). Soak them overnight or at least 5 hours in 3½ cups of cold water.

Place the beans, rice and soaking water in a pressure cooker. Add salt and cook on low flame for 20 minutes. Then raise to high flame until the gauge jiggles.

Place an asbestos pad between the pot and flame. Turn down flame and low cook for 45 - 60 minutes.

Turn the flame off and let pressure return to normal. Remove cover and mix the rice from top to bottom.

Top rice is yin and dry; bottom rice is yang and soft.

Pressure-Cooked Brown Rice 1b.

3 cups brown rice
4½ cups water
½ tsp. sea salt

To wash the rice, place it in a pressure cooker near the sink. Fill a bowl with cool running water and add this to the pressure cooker until the rice is covered with water. Rinse the rice with your hand, stirring from top to bottom. Drain, using a strainer to keep from losing any grains. Repeat this process several times until the rinse water is clear.

Drain the last rinse water and add the measured water. Rice can be left to soak overnight and then cooked in this water.

Cook the rice as in 1a. Wait until cooking to add the salt.

Note: If you have a new pressure cooker, use a 1 to 1 proportion of rice to water.

When cooking 10 or more cups of rice use less water — 10 c. rice, 9 c. water; 25 c. rice, 22 to 23 c. water.

Boiled Brown Rice 1c.

4 cups brown rice
6 cups water
1 tsp. sea salt

Ideally a porcelain-coated cast iron or heavy cast iron pot is best. A stainless steel pot can also be used — the heavier the better.

Rinse the rice gently in a pan with cold water. Keep changing the water and rinsing until the water is clear, as in 1b.

Soak the rice overnight in 6 cups of water.

Add salt just before cooking. Cook on low flame for 30 minutes, then turn flame to high until the boiling point is reached. Cook for 20 minutes on a medium high flame, then 40 minutes on low flame.

Turn flame off and let sit for 20 minutes. Remove the cover and mix the rice thoroughly before serving.

Mochi *(Flour)* 2A.

5 cups sweet brown rice
6 cups water
7 cups sweet brown rice flour

Rinse the rice until the rinse water becomes clear. Soak the rice for 24 hours in a pressure cooker.

Cover and cook using a flame a little higher than medium until it reaches full pressure. Turn flame to low and continue cooking for 20 minutes.

Turn off flame, let pressure return to normal and allow the rice to cool for 45 minutes.

Pound with a suricogi (wooden pestle). Mix in the flour while the rice is very hot and pound it again. Wet both hands in cold water and knead rice, dipping hands into cold water each time before handling the hot rice. When most of the rice grains are broken down, the kneading process is complete.

Bring some water to a boil in a rice steamer. Put a wet cloth into the pan after the water begins to steam. Place the mochi/flour mixture on top of the wet cloth and cover with the cloth. Steam cook in this manner at high heat for 20 minutes.

Pierce the mochi with a dry chopstick; if nothing sticks to it when it is withdrawn, the mochi is done. Spoon out a lump of mochi, form it into a ball and coat it with the covering you prefer.

Steamed Mochi 2B.

7 cups sweet brown rice
4 cups boiling water
6 quart pressure cooker
vegetable steamer with 1½″ legs or base

Wash the sweet rice and soak it 24 hours in about 10 cups of water. Drain and reserve water for soup stock.

Put 4 cups of boiling water in pressure cooker. Set the vegetable steamer in the bottom of the pressure cooker and place the rice on top of the steamer. Cover it and bring the pressure up, using a high flame, until the weight jiggles. Cook the rice for an hour over a medium high flame, allowing weight to jiggle.

Turn off the heat and let pressure return to normal (about 30 min.).

Pour the rice into a large bowl and pound it with a wooden pestle. When the pounded rice cools, steam it for 20 minutes.

Repeat pounding and steaming until the rice grains are completely broken.

Mugwort Mochi 2C.

Follow 2B., steamed mochi or 2A., flour mochi. Add mugwort just before the last pounding. For 7 cups of sweet brown rice, use 5 balls of dried mugwort.

If you use dried mugwort, soak it overnight, boil it for 10 minutes and drain and squeeze it. If you use fresh mugwort, boil it in salted water for a few minutes uncovered over a high flame. Then strain and squeeze off the excess water.

Place it in the center of the pounded mochi. Bring the mochi up around the mugwort to cover it and continue pounding the mochi until the mugwort is evenly mixed with it.

Mochi Soup 2a.

1 med. burdock root, cut sasagaki
2″ of daikon, cut tanzaku
1 carrot, cut sasagaki
3 taro (albi) cut ¼″ koguchigiri
2 scallions, cut ¼″ koguchigiri
7 cups boiling water
½ Tbsp. soy sauce
2 tsp. sesame oil
fresh mochi

Saute the burdock in a covered pan. After 5 minutes stir the burdock with chopsticks dipped in salt and cook 5 minutes more. Repeat this process 2 times. The burdock will begin to smell sweet.

Add the daikon, taro and carrot in that order, sauteeing each before adding the next.

Sprinkle with salt, add boiling water and cook 30 minutes. Add soy sauce and scallions.

Place a spoonful of fresh mochi in a soup bowl, cover it with hot soup and serve it immediately.

Azuki Squash Mochi 2b.

1 cup azuki beans
3 cups water
3 cups sliced winter squash (butternut, Hubbard)
1 tsp. sea salt

Soak azuki beans in 1½ cups of water for at least 5 hours or overnight.

Bring them to a boil on a high flame and add ½ cup of cold water. Repeat this procedure two times. Cook the beans on medium heat until tender (about 1 hour).

Add the sliced squash and salt. Cook until the squash is tender, stirring so that some of it gets mashed, similar to a puree.

This can be served covering fresh mochi or baked on top of the mochi. Serve this dish hot or cold depending on the season.

Walnut Mochi 2c.

2 cups walnuts, slightly roasted
3 Tbsp. soy sauce
3 Tbsp. boiling water

Roast the walnuts until they are slightly brown in color. Grind walnuts into a meal in a suribachi, adding soy sauce and boiling water. Grind ingredients together until they make a butter-like consistency.

Using a wet metal teaspoon, add 1 heaping spoonful of mochi into the walnut mixture. Cover mochi with the walnut meal, and serve.

Baked Mochi with Kinako 2d.

Bake the mochi in an oven at 325 degrees for about 20 minutes. Dip it in amasake (see 8.) and cover it with soybean powder.

Kinako (roasted soybean powder)

Roast soybeans in a dry frying pan over a medium heat until they are slightly browned. When the beans are cooled, grind them in a flour grinder or a blender.

Baked Mochi with Nori 2e.

Bake the mochi in an oven at 325° about 20 minutes or until it is tender. Lightly baste the mochi with tamari soy sauce and cover it with nori (sea weed).

Variation: Mochi can be prepared by heating in a little oil. Use a heavy fry-pan and fry it on both sides about five minutes or until it becomes tender. Be sure to keep mochi covered while frying. Serve with tamari soy sauce or in miso soup.

Lotus Root, Burdock, Carrot, Konnyaku Nishime 3.

½ med. burdock, cut rangiri
1 block konnyaku, cut into 1″ × 2″ squares
2″ lotus root, cut in ⅛ths, then rangiri
1 small carrot, cut in quarters lengthwise, then rangiri
3 tsp. oil
1 Tbsp. tamari soy sauce
¼ tsp. sea salt
8 thin bamboo skewers 5″ long

Heat 1 tsp. oil. Saute the burdock until its smell is gone. Add a little water and cook for 20 minutes. After the liquid begins to boil, add 1 tsp. tamari soy sauce and continue to cook until the burdock is tender.

Cook the lotus root by the same method used for burdock.

Heat 1 tsp. oil and saute the konnyaku well until its bubbles are gone. Add 2 tsp. tamari soy sauce, cover and cook 20 minutes, stirring occasionally.

Add ¼ cup of water to the carrots in a separate pan and bring them to a boil. Lower the flame to medium, cover and cook 10 more minutes.

Add ¼ tsp. salt and cook until the carrots are tender.

Serve on skewers, 2 per person: Lotus root, burdock, konnyaku and carrot.

Kombu, Age, Albi Nishime 4.

10 medium-sized albi
1 tsp. oil
¼ tsp. sea salt
2¼ tsp. tamari soy sauce

Scrub albi and scrape off the outer skin. Heat the oil and saute the whole albi. Add ½ cup cold water and ¼ tsp. tamari soy sauce and boil for 20 minutes.

Add ¼ tsp. salt, 2 tsp. tamari and cook until tender.

1½″ × 24″ piece of kombu
5 pieces home-made age, cut into triangles (see 64.)
1 Tbsp. tamari soy sauce

Soak the kombu in water for 5 minutes. Strain this

water through a clean cotton cloth to remove any sand, and save it. Tie the kombu into knots 3″ apart. Cut leaving 1½″ on either side of knot, and pressure-cook in soaking water for 20 minutes. (If you don't have a pressure cooker, cook it at least 2 hours or until the kombu is tender.)

Add the age and boil for 5 minutes. Add the tamari soy sauce and cook 20 minutes. If there is a lot of water, remove the cover and the excess water will boil away.

Mix and serve kombu, age and albi. Serve 2 albi per person.

This dish is less salty when cold and served on the following day.

Black Bean Nishime 5.

2 cups black beans
4 cups of water
1½ tsp. sea salt

Soak the washed black beans in 4 cups of cold water for one hour.

Bring the beans to a boil in the same water, cover and cook on a low flame for 1½ hours.

Add salt and cook an additional ½ hour over a low flame.

Daikon and Carrot Salad 6.

1 cup daikon, cut very thin sengiri
½ cup carrot, cut same
2 tsp. sea salt

Dressing: 3 Tbsp. orange juice
1 Tbsp. lemon juice
1 tsp. sea salt

Keep the daikon and carrot separate after you have cut them. Mix 1 tsp. of sea salt thoroughly with each vegetable and allow them to sit for 10 minutes.

Place daikon in a strainer and pour 2 cups of boiling water over it. Save this water — it can be used for soup.

Do the same with the carrots.

Let the vegetables drain together and cool. Squeeze off the excess water and mix in the salad dressing.

Allow this to sit overnight, and serve it cool.

Yam-Chestnut Kinton 7.

2 cups sweetmeat squash or yams
2 cups dry chestnuts
1½ tsp. sea salt
1 tsp. minced orange peel

Steam the sliced squash or whole yams and remove the skins while they are still hot. (Note: when using yams, you might try baking at 350° for 1 hour, then peel. This way of cooking makes them sweeter than steamed.)

Add ½ tsp. salt and mash.

Wash the chestnuts and cover them with ½″ of warm water for 2 hours (or overnight, in cold water).

Cook until chestnuts are half done — about 30 minutes. Add the remaining salt, finish cooking, drain the excess liquid and set them aside to cool.

Mix the whole cooled chestnuts with the mashed yam or squash and boil this uncovered for 10 minutes or until the mixture is thick, like mashed potatoes.

Stir in the orange peel and remove from heat. Serve cold.

This is like a pudding.

Amasake 8.

Amasake can be made from sweet brown rice, barley, wheat, millet or any grain.

2 cups sweet brown rice
4 cups water
¼ cup koji (malt yeast culture)

Rinse the rice gently in a pan of cold water, changing the water until it is clear. Soak overnight in 4 cups of water.

Pressure cook the rice on a flame slightly higher than medium until the pressure comes up. Turn down to low flame and cook for 20 minutes. Turn off flame and let rice stand for 45 minutes.

When it is cool enough to hold in hands, mix the warm rice with the koji in a glass or porcelain bowl and allow it to ferment 3 - 4 hours. DO NOT USE A METAL BOWL. Keep this rice and koji mixture covered and in a warm place. During the fermentation period, mix the rice top to bottom several times until the koji has disappeared or melted.

Then put the mixture in a pan and heat it on a medium flame. Turn flame off as soon as one or two bubbles appear to indicate the boiling stage. Allow the mixture to cool again and put in a glass jar in the refrigerator. Amasake can be eaten 5 - 7 days later.

To obtain a smoother texture, amasake can be blended. It can be kept longer in a cold place. It can be cooked over a low flame until it is slightly brown. Do not use a cover while cooking it.

Amasake is very sweet and can be used to sweeten cakes, karinto (fried dough cake), doughnuts, cookies and pies. To serve amasake as a warm drink, add boiling water and salt, bring to a boil and serve.

Note: For cakes, cookies and doughnuts use 1 cup sweet brown rice and 1 cup of koji.

Amasake Kanten 8a.

1 cup amasake concentrate or 1 cup yinnie syrup
4 cups tangerine juice
6 cups water
2 heaping Tbsp. kanten powder or 2 kanten bars
2 tsp. sea salt

Dissolve the kanten in cold water and boil it for 20 minutes with salt in an uncovered pot.

Add the amasake concentrate and cook 5 more minutes. Remove the pot from the stove and let it cool to room temperature, then add the tangerine juice. Don't boil the tangerine juice — this causes it to lose its flavor. Mix well.

Rinse a jello bowl or square cookie sheet with cold water. Add the kanten mixture and chill it.

Tazukuri with Yinnie Syrup 9.

2 cups tazukuri (small dried blue fish)
2 Tbsp. tamari soy sauce
2 Tbsp. Japanese sake
1 Tbsp. yinnie syrup

Roast the tazukuri in a dry skillet until they are well dried and brownish in color.

In another pan mix the tamari soy sauce, yinnie syrup and sake. Cook them together uncovered over a low flame for 5 minutes or until the mixture becomes thick. Add the roasted fish and shake the pan until the sauce covers the fish. Place them in a dish to cool.

Yinnies are good with this crispy fish dish.

Baked Fish with Salt 10.

3 lbs. whole fish (such as mackerel or bass)
1 Tbsp. fresh ginger juice
2 Tbsp. sea salt

Clean the fish, removing the scales and internal organs. Make 2 deep diagonal cuts to the bone on both sides of the fish. Cover the entire fish with ginger juice and 1 Tbsp. of salt and let it sit 1 hour.

Wipe all of the salt off the fish with a paper towel (this takes away some of the fish smell) and place the fish in a baking pan or on a cookie sheet. From a height of about 1 foot sprinkle the remaining 1 Tbsp. of salt on the sides of the fish. This will give it a nice white glaze when it is baked.

Place the fish in a preheated oven and bake it 45 minutes to 1 hour at 450°.

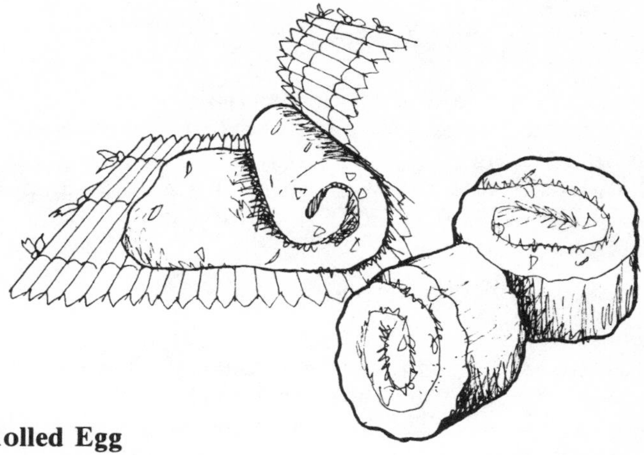

Rolled Egg 11.

1 egg
½ cup unbleached white flour
½ cup water
½ cup cooked squash (acorn or sweetmeat)
1 tsp. sea salt

Mix the flour and water and add the beaten egg. Add steamed squash from which the skins have been removed. Add 1 tsp. salt.

Heat a little oil in a skillet, pour the egg mixture into the heated skillet and brown it slightly on both sides (about 5 minutes) on a medium flame.

Remove the omelette and set it on a bamboo mat which you have placed on a cutting board. Roll the omelette into a square or round shape like a sushi roll. Leave the mat around the omelette until the shape is set and it is cool.

Cut it into straight or diagonal slices ½″ thick.

Bancha *(Twig)* Tea 12.

Bancha is a roasted three-year-old green tea that contains the leaves and small twigs of the tea bush. It aids in removing toxins from the body in the case of persons who have taken drugs; it also aids the body in producing Vitamin C. It is good for children and contains no caffeine.

Preparing Tea

To prepare, dry roast the leaves in a pan over a medium flame for a few minutes. Stir constantly to prevent burning. Pick out the twigs and pour the leaves into a clean glass jar after cooling. Dry roast the twigs a second time until they turn brown, then mix. Unroasted tea leaves can be used, but roasted leaves provide more flavor.

Making Tea

Add ¼ cup of tea leaves to 4 - 6 cups of boiling water. Turn off the flame and let the leaves steep for a few minutes before serving. When the liquid is all gone, add more water and boil ten minutes. Add a teaspoon of fresh leaves and let tea steep a few minutes before serving. This process can be repeated until the leaves form a layer one inch deep in the bottom of the tea pot.

Note: When making all teas, glass or porcelain pots should be used for best results.

Old leaves can be used for compost, or saved for making koi-koku (carp soup) with dry tea leaves.

Natto with Pickled Daikon Leaves 13.

1 4-oz. pkg. of natto (available in Japanese stores, or see 73. or 73a. for home-made natto)
1 daikon top pickled in nuka (see 14.)
pinch of sea salt
2 - 3 tsp. tamari soy sauce

Wash the daikon tops well, squeeze out the water and chop them finely. Add salt to the natto and mix it well. Thread-like strands will appear as you mix. Add the tamari soy sauce and mix it in well. Then add the daikon tops and mix again.

Note: Natto is fermented soy beans. It is a high-quality protein and is good for aiding digestion.

Daikon Nuka Pickles 14.

Step 1: 5 gallon crock or tamari keg
30 - 40 daikon the size of your lower arm
1 cup sea salt

Wash the daikon, separate the leaves and the roots. Let these drain for ½ day.

Place a handful of salt in the bottom of the crock and put in a layer of daikon root. Fill in any spaces with daikon leaves until all is tightly packed. Spread a handful of salt on this layer; repeat layerings until all the daikon is used. You will have about 3 - 4 layers.

Place daikon leaves on the top layer, sprinkle the last handful of salt on the leaves and then place a wooden lid and 15 lb. stone on top. Cover the keg with plastic — be sure to tie this plastic cover on.

After 4 days water will cover the top of the vegetables. Take all the daikon out of the crock. Remove and boil the remaining salted water and save it. If you are making pickles and not enough water has come out of the vegetables to cover them, add this reserved water; otherwise the vegetables will spoil.

Step 2: 1 cup sea salt
14 heaping cups roasted rice bran (nuka)
1 cup currants

Mix the rice bran and salt together. Place a handful of this mixture on the bottom of the crock. Add a layer of prepared daikon (see Step 1.). Sprinkle over the daikon 2 handfuls of the mixture and add 1 handful of currants.

Repeat these layers, using daikon leaves to tightly fill the empty spaces. Use daikon leaves to cover the top. Place a wooden lid and 15 lb. stone on top and tie a plastic cover over the keg.

If after 1 week there is no water covering the pickles, add 4 cups of your reserved salt water. Remove the stone and lid, pour this water around the inside edge of the crock, and replace stone and lid. This will pull the water out of the vegetables overnight.

When water covers the daikon, remove the stone for 24 hours. All the liquid will go to the bottom. Keep a 5 lb. stone on top for pressure. The water should be covering the daikon. These daikon will be ready to eat in 3 weeks.

Daikon leaves are very nutritious. Wash them well, chop and mix with tamari soy sauce and use as a condiment with grain. Mixed with natto and tamari and served with grain, these pickles are very sweet.

Variation: 1 cup of dates, raisins or prunes can be placed between the layers to make a flavorful sweet pickle. Place ½ cup persimmon skin or 2 - 3 tangerine rinds on top of the daikon leaves. When the water comes, remove and discard them.

Chinese Cabbage Nuka Pickles 15.

20 lbs. Chinese cabbage (about 6 - 7 heads)
5 cups nuka (rice bran)
1 cup sea salt
1 3″× 12″ piece of dashi (thick) kombu cut in 1″ pieces

Wash the cabbage. Remove and save the outer green leaves from each head. Quarter each head of cabbage by cutting about 2″ down at the core of the head and breaking the cabbage apart with your fingers. If the core is thick, make two 2″ cuts into the core.

Dry the cabbage in the shade outside for half a day.

Roast the nuka. When it is cool, mix in a handful of sea salt. Place the mixture on the bottom of the keg. Cover this with half of the outer green leaves which you have removed. Sprinkle each piece of cabbage on the inside with about 1 tsp. salt and place them tightly in the keg. Alternate the direction of each layer, placing a few strips of kombu between the layers.

On top of everything, place the remaining outer green leaves and the remaining salt. Place a 10 - 20 lb. stone weight on top of a wooden cover until water comes out of the vegetables (about 2 - 3 days).

Then change the pressure to about 5 lbs. You can eat these pickles in about 7 days.

The cabbage pickles need not be washed since the nuka is in contact with the outer green leaves only. The outer green leaves can be eaten. Wash the nuka off, chop them up finely and add raw chopped scallions, bonita flakes and a bit of soy sauce. Mix these thoroughly and sprinkle over rice.

Keep pickles stored in a cool, shady spot.

Chinese cabbage prepared in this way is delicious and rich in minerals.

Buckwheat Noodles with Clear Soup 16.

1 lb. buckwheat noodles (soba)
3″ × 6″ dashi kombu
1 sheet nori (see 16b.)
3 scallions, cut hasugiri
1 heaping Tbsp. tempura crumbs (see 22c.)
7 chuba iriko (dried fish)
1 tsp. sea salt
3 Tbsp. tamari soy sauce

Add the kombu to 3 cups of cold water and bring to a boil. Add the fish, boil again and strain. Reserve the stock.

Add 3 cups of cold water to the kombu and fish and boil it for 20 minutes. Strain and reserve the second stock and mix it with the first.

Take 3 cups of this soup stock, add 2 cups cold water and salt and boil 20 minutes. Add the tempura crumbs and continue to boil the stock, adding the scallions and tamari soy sauce to taste.

Bring 8 cups of cold water to a boil and add buckwheat noodles. When the liquid returns to a boil add 1 cup of cold water and cover. After the liquid boils a third time, turn off the flame and let it sit a few minutes. Then stir the noodles, mixing the bottom with the top.

To see if the noodles are ready, take one noodle, rinse it under cold water and cut it. If the inside and outside are the same color, the noodles are done. If not, boil them once more.

Strain the noodles and serve them with the hot soup. If you wish to serve cold noodles, rinse with cold water until they are cool.

Chick Pea Sauce 17.

1 cup chick peas
2 med. onions, 1 cut mijingiri, the other ¼″ mawashigiri
1 med. carrot, cut ¼″ sainome
10 cabbage leaves, cut into 1″ squares
1 stalk of celery, cut ¼″ hasugiri
2 tsp. sea salt
1 Tbsp. sesame butter
1 tsp. sesame oil
Boiling water

Wash and soak the chick peas in 2 cups of water overnight or at least 5 hours, in a pressure cooker. Bring to pressure and cook 45 minutes on a low flame. Let pressure come down to normal and remove the cover.

Heat the oil in another pan, saute the onions (cut mijingiri) until they are slightly brown in color, then add the other onions and saute until they are transparent.

Add the cabbage, celery and then the carrots, sauteeing each until the color changes before adding the next vegetable. Add boiling water to cover vegetables and bring them to a boil on a high flame. Cook this 20 minutes on a medium flame.

Add the chick peas without stirring. Sprinkle in the salt and continue to cook until everything is tender. Stir and add the sesame butter, which has been diluted with some of the liquid from the cooking vegetables. Cook for 5 minutes more.

If more salt is needed, add tamari soy sauce to taste.

Vegetable Miso Soup 18.

1 med. onion, cut thin mawashigiri
2 med. turnips, cut bite-size ¼″ thick
½ carrot, cut sengiri
1 tsp. sesame oil
6 cups boiling water
1 heaping Tbsp. mugi (barley) miso

Heat the oil and saute the onions until they are transparent. Add the turnips and saute them until their color changes, then add the carrots and saute a few minutes more. Add boiling water and turn flame to high. Remove the cover and cook for a few minutes. This removes the excess oil and the strong flavors of the vegetables.

With the cover on, cook on a medium flame for 45 minutes or until the vegetables are tender.

Place the miso into a strainer. Turn off the flame under the soup and add the miso by mashing it through the strainer. Then invert the strainer and place all of the contents into the soup.

Note: All miso soup vegetables must be bite-size and completely cooked.

Collard Green, Onion, Carrot, Celery Nitsuke 19.

1 bunch collard greens, cut 1″ koguchigiri
2 med. onions, cut thin mawashigiri
1 small carrot, cut sasagaki
2 stalks of celery, cut thin hasugiri
1 Tbsp. oil
½ tsp. sea salt
1 Tbsp. tamari soy sauce

Saute the onions until they are transparent. Add the collard greens and cook them until they are bright green. Add the celery, then the carrot. Saute a few minutes and add the tamari at the same time. Cook with a cover on a low flame for 5 minutes. Turn the flame to medium and cook for 20 minutes or until the vegetables are tender.

Serve this hot.

Mackerel with Ginger Miso 20.

5 large pieces of mackerel
3 Tbsp. barley (mugi) miso
1½ cups water
1 tsp. grated ginger

Soften the miso in water. Bring it to a boil and add the ginger.

Add the fish and cook without a cover on a medium flame for 10 minutes on one side. Then turn it over and cook it on the other side for 10 minutes.

Serve the fish hot with the sauce.

Tossed Salad 21a.

½ head of lettuce (torn into 1″ squares)
1 medium cucumber, cut thin hangetsugiri
½ cup grapes
1 small tomato, cut ¼″ mawashigiri
1 hard-boiled egg (yolk grated, white cut mijingiri)
1 dill pickle, cut ¼″ ichogiri

Take the cucumber and cut ½″ off the stem. Cover the cut surfaces with salt and rub them together to take away any bitter taste in the cucumber.

Wash and cut ingredients according to directions above. Mix the lettuce, cucumber, grapes, dill pickle and egg white together thoroughly.

Decorate the top with the tomato slices and the grated egg yolk.

Note: The grapes, egg, dill pickle and tomato are optional items. For more variety you can add watermelon rind cut in ½″ cubes. This recipe is for summer use. For winter it is better to substitute winter vegetables like lettuce, celery and carrots.

Salad Dressing 21b.

2 Tbsp. corn oil
1 Tbsp. lemon juice
3 Tbsp. orange juice
1 Tbsp. minced onion
2 tsp. sea salt

Heat the oil, then allow it to cool.

Beat the oil, salt, lemon juice and orange juice together until the color becomes cloudy. Add the minced onion and mix well.

Wait 20 minutes before adding it to the tossed salad.

Assorted Vegetable Tempura 22a.

1 cup whole wheat pastry flour
1¼ cups cold water
½ tsp. sea salt
1 heaping tsp. arrowroot starch
5 string beans, cut thin hasugiri
1 med. onion, cut thin mawashigiri
1″ of carrot, cut thin sengiri
oil for tempura (corn and safflower)

Mix the dry ingredients, add a cup of water and mix. Add the remaining ¼ cup of water and mix vigorously. The batter may remain slightly lumpy.

Mix half safflower and half corn oil, about 3″ deep in a cast iron pan, and heat the oil. To test the oil temperature, sprinkle some salt and listen for a sizzling sound. Or drop a little batter into the oil. If the oil is hot enough, it will immediately rise to the top. Turn the flame off for 1 minute.

Mix the vegetables and batter together and drop them by teaspoonfuls into the oil. If they fall apart, the batter is too watery. Turn the flame to high. When the batter is slightly golden, turn the vegetables over and fry them until both sides are a golden color.

Place the tempura in a strainer set in a pan to catch the excess oil. Just before the next batch of tempura is ready, remove the previous batch from the strainer and place on paper towels. Repeat until all tempura is cooked.

Note: When the oil has cooled and is only slightly warm, put it into a glass bottle to save.

Use absorbent cotton on the strainer to remove leftover particles. This oiled cotton can be used to oil bread pans, etc.

Tempura 22b.

1 cup whole wheat pastry flour
2 Tbsp. rice flour
1¼ cup water
1 tsp. sea salt
2 tsp. arrowroot starch
1 small egg
oil for tempura

Beat the egg, salt and water together. Mix the flour into the water with two thick chopsticks. The batter may remain slightly lumpy.

Heat the oil. It should be at least 3″ deep. Stir it with chopsticks so the temperature is uniform. When it begins to smolder (about 330°) test to see if a drop of batter rises to the top or if there is a "sputter" sound when a bit of salt is added. If so, the oil is ready.

If the oil is too shallow or too many pieces are dropped in at once the temperature will fall quickly and tempura will become oily. Tempura floating freely in oil will be crispy. Poor quality oil evaporates quickly and burns easily.

When the tempura turns a light golden color, turn over and cook until both sides are the same color. Place the tempura in a strainer set in a pan to catch the excess oil. Remove the tempura to paper towels before the next batch is ready to drain.

The following foods I serve according to the season.

Warm weather tempura

Yam or sweet potato: cut these like French fries.
Eggplant: slice into pieces ¼″ thick.
Potato: the same as for the yam.
Summer squash: cut into strips 1″ × 3″ × ¼″.
Green pepper: slice in rounds ¼″ thick and remove the seeds.
Celery leaves: use the leafy section 5″ long; dip only one side into batter.
Shiso leaves: same as celery.
Asparagus: cut into pieces 3½″ long from the tip and dip into batter.
Scallions: cut into 1½″ lengths.
Nori: cut in half lengthwise and then into 5 strips widthwise; dip each strip halfway into batter, or on one side only.

Cold weather tempura

Carrot: cut into ¼″ rounds on the diagonal.
Burdock: cut on the diagonal 5″ long and ⅛″ thick.
Onion: slice into rounds ¼″ thick.
Winter squash: cut into strips 1″ × 3″ and ½″ × ¼″.
Carrot greens: use the leafy section 5″ long; dip only one side into batter.
Cauliflower: use flowerettes 3″ long.
Broccoli: the same as cauliflower.
Shrimp or prawns: remove the skin but leave the tail on. Slice across the ends of the tail and squeeze out the water. Slit the back of the prawns and remove the intestines. Make 3 short lateral cuts on the short side of the prawn to straighten it. Dip in batter while holding the tail.
Abalone: pound it gently and cut into slices ¼″ thick and 3″ wide.
Squid: remove the skin and cut into pieces 1½″ × 3½″.

Grated ginger can be served with fish tempura dishes.

Tempura Crumbs 22c.

Take the leftover tempura batter and drop ⅓ cup at a time into hot oil. Scramble with chopsticks. Let the pieces brown slightly on both sides, turning them once in a while.

Strain and reserve the excess oil. When it is cool, put in a glass jar or container for future use.

Tempura crumbs are very useful in noodle soup and vegetable nitsuke. They can be stored in the refrigerator.

Tempura Sauce 22d.

1 cup soup stock (see 16.)
¼ cup tamari soy sauce

Bring these ingredients to a boil, then allow to cool. Serve it in small individual dishes.

Add grated daikon and/or carrot to each serving as desired.

Grated Daikon and Carrot 23.

1″ of daikon, grated
1″ of carrot, grated

Mix the vegetables together or place the carrot on top of daikon. Serve with tamari soy sauce.

Grated daikon is usually served with tempura, as daikon aids in digesting oily foods. Equal amounts of grated carrot and grated daikon mixed together will please the children — it is milder and more colorful.

Kasha 24.

1½ cups kasha (roasted)
1 medium onion, cut mijingiri
2″ of carrot, cut mijingiri
3 cups cold water
1 tsp. sesame oil
1 tsp. sea salt

Heat the oil. Saute the onions until they are transparent. Add the carrot, cover and cook, periodically stirring until the carrots are tender.

Add the kasha and saute a few minutes. Add 1½ cups of cold water and bring the mixture to a boil. Add the remaining water and boil on a low flame for 30 - 45 minutes.

An asbestos pad will keep this dish from burning.

Sesame Onion Sauce 25.

1 med. onion, cut mijingiri
½ tsp. sesame oil
1 heaping Tbsp. sesame butter
2 - 3 Tbsp. tamari soy sauce
1½ cups boiling water

Heat the oil. Saute the onions until they are slightly brown in color. Add water, bring to a boil and cook for 20 minutes on a medium flame.

Add sesame butter which has been diluted and softened with a little warm water. Cook this for a few minutes. Add tamari soy sauce and cook a few minutes more.

Serve the sauce with chopped parsley or watercress.

Boiled Beets 26.

2 med. beets, roots cut ¼″ mawashigiri, leaves cut 1½″ koguchigiri
½ cup water

Cook the beets in water for 20 minutes on a medium flame in a covered pot. Add the leaves and cook these until they are tender. Add more water if necessary.

Note: Umeboshi pits cooked with beets bring out the taste.

Azuki Chestnut Kanten 27.

1 cup azuki beans
1 cup dried chestnuts
1 tsp. sea salt
2 bars kanten
8½ cups water

Soak the azuki beans and chestnuts together overnight in 3 cups of water.

Bring them to a boil, add ½ cup of cold water. Boil again and add ½ cup cold water. Repeat this once more.

Cook the beans 1 hour until they are tender. Add ½ tsp. sea salt and cook for 20 minutes more.

Wash the kanten bars and break them into small pieces. Soak them for 20 minutes in 4 cups of cold water. Add remaining salt and cook the kanten 20 minutes in an uncovered pot. Add the cooked azuki/chestnut mixture and cook 15 minutes more, still uncovered, stirring frequently.

Place this in a square glass baking dish and allow to cool. When it is firm, remove it from the dish and invert. The bottom will be glistening and shiny. Cut and serve.

Variation: ½ cup yinnie syrup or ½ cup currants, dates or raisins may be substituted for the dried chestnuts.

Wakame Miso Soup 28.

1 med. onion, cut thin mawashigiri
4 3″ strips of wakame, cut ½″ koguchigiri
1 heaping Tbsp. barley miso
5 cups water
1 tsp. sesame oil

Soak the wakame by covering it with cold water for 5-10 minutes. Strain and place it in a bowl filled with water. Shake-wash and drain it again. Strain the soaking water through a fine cotton cloth and reserve for soup stock.

Remove the hard part of the wakame and chop it up finely. The softer part is cut into ½″ pieces.

Heat the oil and saute the onion until transparent. Add water and the finely chopped wakame and bring this to a boil on a high flame. Add the soft part of the wakame and continue boiling on a medium flame for 20 minutes or until the vegetables are tender.

Measure the miso and place it in a strainer. Turn off the flame and place the strainer in the soup. Using a wooden spoon or suricogi, press the miso through the strainer. Whatever will not press through, put into the soup. Serve immediately.

Note: Miso soup is good for removing nicotine from the body. Wakame miso soup is a blood purifier.

Pan-Fried Whole Wheat Spaghetti with Vegetables 29.

1 8-oz. pkg. whole wheat spaghetti
2 med. onions, cut thin mawashigiri
1 small head cabbage, cut thin sengiri
2 stalks celery, cut thin hasugiri
1 Tbsp. sesame oil
2 Tbsp. corn oil
1½ tsp. sea salt
2 Tbsp. tamari soy sauce

Bring 8 cups of water to a boil and add 1 heaping tsp. salt. Sprinkle the spaghetti into the pot, stir with chopsticks and cover. Bring the spaghetti to a boil on a high flame, add one cup of cold water and bring to a boil again. Turn heat off and let sit for 1 minute. Strain and wash the spaghetti in cold water. Drain off the excess water and save it for bread-making (be sure to adjust the salt content for the bread recipe).

Heat the oil in a pan over a high flame and saute the onions until slightly transparent. Add the cabbage and celery and saute until their color becomes bright. Add remaining salt, stir and cook vegetables a few minutes longer.

Heat another cast iron pot or a wok and add 2 Tbsp. of corn oil. When the oil is heated, add the spaghetti. Press down, cover and cook on a medium high flame for 7 minutes or until spaghetti appears light brown in color. Turn and cook another 7 minutes, covered. Turn once more and then shut off the flame.

Add tamari soy sauce by sprinkling it around the edges. Let this sit covered for a few minutes, then stir.

Spaghetti and vegetables can be mixed together and served, or the vegetables can be placed on top of the spaghetti.

Nori Nitsuke 30.

1 package nori
2 cups water
2 - 3 Tbsp. tamari soy sauce

Tear nori into 1″ squares and soak it in the water for 20 minutes.

Boil it on a medium flame in the same water for 20 minutes. Add tamari soy sauce and cook for 20 minutes longer, covered.

If the nori is too watery remove the cover and cook until the extra liquid evaporates.

Apple Pie 31.

Crust:
3 cups whole wheat pastry flour
3 Tbsp. oil
1 cup cold water

Filling:
5 med. apples, cut in 8 pieces, then ¼″ thick
½ tsp. sea salt
2 Tbsp. arrowroot flour
6 Tbsp. water
1 tsp. cinnamon

Mix the oil and whole wheat flour by rubbing with your fingers so that there are no lumps. Add cold water and mix with a fork. Be careful not to knead the dough.

In another bowl mix the arrowroot with water. Be sure it dissolves completely, then add the cinnamon, salt and

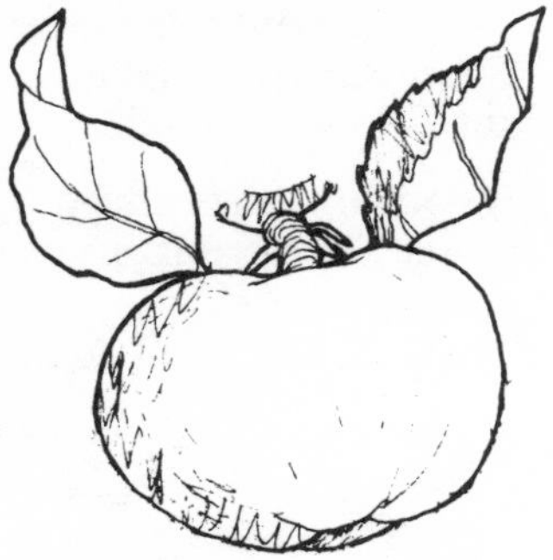

finally the apples.

Divide the pie crust dough in half and roll one of the halves into a circle. This should be ½″ more than the diameter of the pie pan. Oil the pie pan. Fold the dough in half, then in quarters. Center the corner in the pie pan, then spread the dough out and trim around the edge of the pie pan.

Put in the apple mixture. Roll out the other half of the pie dough and cover the pie. Press the edges together and make a design of your own at the seam. Cut a cross in the center for steam to escape.

Bake the pie at 450° for 45 minutes or until it is slightly brown on top.

To glaze the crust for special occasions, brush the top with a beaten egg.

Note: Whole wheat pastry flour can be substituted for arrowroot flour — it has a sweeter taste. Also, by slicing apples thicker you don't need as many as when they are thinly sliced.

Kidney Beans with Miso 32.

1½ cups kidney beans
3 cups cold water
1 Tbsp. mugi miso (barley miso)
2″ × 2″ dashi kombu

Wash the beans and soak them overnight or at least 5 hours.

Place them in a pressure cooker with kombu and cook for 45 minutes. Turn off the heat, let pressure come down and remove the lid. Add the miso and stir gently. Cook for 30 - 45 minutes covered and without pressure on a low flame.

Note: Legumes seasoned with miso provide balanced protein and proper salt proportions.

Vegetable Stew with Sake 33.

5 small whole turnips
3 med. onions, cut in quarters
1 carrot, cut thick hasugiri, 5 pieces
1 stalk celery, cut ¼″ hasugiri
6 cups boiling water
1 Tbsp. oil
½ cup bechamel sauce (see 37a.)
2 tsp. sea salt
2 Tbsp. sake

Saute the onions until they are transparent. Add the turnips, saute about 7 minutes and then add the carrot and celery. When the celery becomes bright green in color, add the boiling water and cook for 20 minutes. Add the salt and cook the stew 20 minutes more or until all the vegetables are tender.

Mix the bechamel sauce with 1 cup of cold water and add it to the vegetables to thicken them. If necessary, add soy sauce to season.

Add the sake, bring to a boil and serve immediately.

Winter Squash and Onion Nitsuke 34.

1 small Hokkaido squash or any winter squash, cut in 1½″ squares
3 med. onions, cut mawashigiri
1 Tbsp. oil
½ tsp. sea salt
1 Tbsp. tamari soy sauce
⅓ cup boiling water

Saute the onions. When they become transparent, add the squash and saute 5 minutes. Add salt and tamari soy sauce. Cover the pan and cook on a low flame for 10 minutes.

If no water comes, add the boiling water around the edge of the pan and cook the nitsuke 25 minutes or until the squash is tender.

Onion Miso 35.

5 med. onions, cut ¼″ mawashigiri
2 - 3 Tbsp. used oil
2 heaping Tbsp. barley miso

Heat the oil and saute the onions until they are transparent. Cover the pot and cook until the onions are tender. They will be very soft and have some dark spots.

Spread the miso over the onions, cover and cook for 5 minutes more. Then stir the mixture. If it is watery, cook uncovered until there is less liquid.

Note: This dish is good for heart and lung diseases. For anemic and sick people, be sure to use sesame oil. This dish tastes good on hot cereal.

Vegetable Gratin 36.

8 cabbage leaves
1 bunch of broccoli
2 med. carrots
2 med. onions, cut ¼″ mawashigiri
1 tsp. sesame oil
1 tsp. sea salt
½ cup bechamel sauce (37a.)
2 heaping Tbsp. bread crumbs

Bring 4 cups of water to a boil and add 1 heaping tsp. of salt. Cook the cabbage leaves, broccoli stems, carrots and broccoli flowerettes, in that order. Use bamboo skewer to test the vegetables to see if they are tender. Remove vegetables.

Place 4 cabbage leaves together, roll them very tightly and cut into 1″ pieces. Repeat with remaining cabbage leaves. Cut the carrots in 1½″ koguchigiri style. Cut the broccoli stems in ½″ koguchigiri. The flowerettes remain whole.

Heat the oil and saute the onions. Cover and stir them occasionally until they are tender.

Make a bechamel sauce from the water used to cook the vegetables. Place the sauteed onions on the bottom of a casserole dish, arrange the cabbage, carrot and broccoli on top of the onions, and cover them with the bechamel sauce. Sprinkle on bread crumbs.

Cook the gratin in a pre-heated oven at 400° for 40 minutes. When the bechamel sauce bubbles, it is done.

Variation: Use Brussels sprouts, cauliflower, celery or leftover vegetable nitsuke or croquettes.

Bechamel Sauce 37.

1 cup whole wheat pastry flour
1 Tbsp. sesame oil
2 - 3 tsp. sea salt
2 cups cold water
1 cup boiling water

Heat the oil and saute the flour on medium-low flame until it is fragrant. Allow it to cool.

Mix 2 cups of cold water with the cooled, roasted flour. Then add boiling water and stir. Add salt and bring the sauce to a boil. Cook it uncovered for 20 minutes on a low flame.

Note: If you have no time to cool the roasted flour, place the pan in cold water in the sink. It is better to use a heavy iron frying pan since this keeps an even temperature.

Onion Sake Bechamel Sauce 37a.

1 med. onion, chopped fine
1 Tbsp. oil
1 cup roasted bechamel sauce (37.)
6 cups water
2 tsp. sea salt
2 Tbsp. sake

Saute the onion in oil until it is transparent. Then add water and cook for 20 minutes. Add salt.

Add cold water to the bechamel sauce, thinning it slightly, then add this to the onions. Cook this sauce for 20 minutes. Add the sake and boil it again. Serve.

Kasha Croquettes 38.

2 cups cooked kasha (see 24.)
½ cup whole wheat pastry flour
1 tsp. sea salt
⅓ cup sweet rice flour
2 Tbsp. corn oil

Mix the cooked kasha with the flour and salt. Shape this dough into croquettes and dust them with sweet rice flour.

Heat the oil in a pan and cook the croquettes on a medium flame for 7 minutes. Turn them over and cook uncovered until they are slightly browned on the bottom.

Sweet rice flour makes a white spot on the croquettes — it is beautiful.

Lettuce Goma Ai *(Cooked Salad)* 39.

15 outer lettuce leaves, whole
1 heaping tsp. sea salt
1 heaping Tbsp. sesame butter or tahini
2 Tbsp. tamari soy sauce
4 cups water

Bring the water to a boil with the salt. Add the washed lettuce leaves and boil without a cover. Turn the leaves over in the pot and boil them again.

Remove the leaves and place them in a strainer to cool. When they are completely cool, squeeze out the excess water. Cut them in 1″ koguchigiri.

Mix the sesame butter and soy sauce together and add this mixture to the lettuce.

Variation: Chinese cabbage or any leafy green vegetables can be used in this recipe.

Russian Soup 40.

½ cup roasted brown rice
5 small whole onions
5 small whole turnips
2 med. carrot, cut on diagonal in 1″ pieces
1 Tbsp. oil
½ cup bechamel sauce (see 37.)
8 cups boiling water
3 - 4 tsp. sea salt
1 Tbsp. minced parsley
turkey giblets (optional)

Saute the onions until they are transparent. Add the turnips, carrot and rice, sauteeing each for a few minutes. Add boiling water and cook the soup for 1 hour. Add salt and cook for as long as possible. If you are using turkey giblets, add these after adding the boiling water.

Thirty minutes before serving, add the bechamel sauce and seasoning to taste. Sprinkle with parsley and serve.

Variation: Quail or chicken bones may also be used to flavor this soup.

Baked Brown Rice 41.

2 cups brown rice
4 cups boiling water
½ tsp. sea salt

Wash the rice the same as 1b. Drain the last rinsing water thoroughly. Roast the rice in a dry skillet over a medium flame until it is golden brown in color.

Place the roasted rice with the salt in a casserole and cover it with boiling water. Bake it at 350° for 1 hour in a covered casserole.

This rice will be light and fluffy, quite different from pressure-cooked rice. It is easier to digest and good for children, older people and those with weight problems.

Variation: This rice can be roasted in a small amount of oil and mixed with sauteed onions, carrots and celery. Whole dried peas, soaked for 5 hours, can be baked with the rice. If you use fresh peas, about 1 cup, they should be added to the rice about 5 minutes before the end of the cooking time. Shrimp or chicken can be mixed with baked rice for another variation.

Prune Kanten 42.

1 lb. prunes (pitted)
6 cups water
1 heaping Tbsp. kanten powder or 2 kanten bars
1 tsp. sea salt

Soak the prunes in 4 cups of water for 1 hour.

Dissolve the kanten and salt in 2 cups of water. Add the prunes and the soaking water and cook 20 minutes uncovered.

Pour this into a mold and let it cool. When the kanten is firm, slice and serve it.

Burdock, Carrot, Lotus Root Kinpira 43.

2 med. burdock, cut sengiri
3 carrots, cut sengiri
1″ of lotus root, cut ichogiri
1 Tbsp. oil
½ tsp. sea salt
2 Tbsp. tamari soy sauce
½ cup boiling water

Saute the burdock in a covered pan. After 5 minutes dip a wooden cooking spoon in some salt and stir the burdock. Let cook 5 minutes more with a cover on. Repeat this process 2 times — the burdock will have a sweet smell.

Add the carrot and then the lotus root. Add the salt, tamari soy sauce and water at the same time. Cook this on a medium flame, covered, until it is tender — about 35 minutes. Add more water if necessary.

Boiled Chinese Cabbage 44.

1 medium whole Chinese cabbage, cut in quarters
1 heaping Tbsp. sea salt
6 cups water

Bring the water to a boil with the sea salt. Use a tall thin pot like a coffee pot or an asparagus cooker. Place the Chinese cabbage in the pot with the core at the bottom. Bring it to a boil uncovered and boil for 5 minutes.

Test the tenderness of the vegetable with a bamboo skewer; when the cabbage is done, place it in a strainer, cool and squeeze out the excess water. Remove the core and slice it 1″ koguchigiri.

Serve the cabbage cool or warm.

Rice Loaf 45.

2 cups cooked brown rice
10 cups whole wheat flour
3 cups brown rice flour
1 Tbsp. sea salt

Mix all of the above ingredients and allow them to sit overnight at room temperature.

Divide into 3 loaves and place each loaf in an oiled bread pan. Place them in the oven for 1 hour with just the pilot light on.

Then bake them at 250° for 2 hours.

Variation: Use bean flour or any other grain flour. Determine your own proportion, but always use twice that amount of whole wheat flour.

Burdock, Carrot and Lotus Root with Oily Miso 46.

½ cup lotus root, cut ichogiri
½ cup burdock, cut sasagaki
½ cup carrot, cut sasagaki
1 cup onion, cut thin mawashigiri
½ cup barley miso
¼ cup boiling water (if necessary)
3 Tbsp. sesame oil
bit of sea salt

Saute the burdock in sesame oil in a covered pan. After 5 minutes, dip chopsticks or wooden spoon in salt. Stir the burdock, cook 5 minutes more and add a pinch of salt. Repeat this process 2 times — the burdock will begin to smell sweet.

Add the onion and cook uncovered until the onion is transparent. Add the carrot and lotus root, then cover and cook the vegetables for 10 minutes. If the burdock is still hard, add boiling water around the edge of the pan and cook 20 minutes more.

When the burdock is soft, cover the vegetables with the miso but don't mix them. Cook 5 minutes covered; steam will make the miso soft. Then stir and mix the miso with the vegetables and cook uncovered until the miso has a fragrant smell.

This is a good dish for a cold winter day. It helps warm the body and creates a hearty appetite.

Cauliflower with Kuzu Sauce 47.

1 med. cauliflower
3 med. onions, cut ¼″ mawashigiri
1 med. carrot, cut rangiri
2 stalks celery, cut ¼″ hasugiri
1 heaping Tbsp. kuzu or arrowroot flour, dissolved in ½ cup cold water
½ tsp. sea salt
2 - 3 Tbsp. tamari
1 Tbsp. sesame oil
5 cups boiling water

Separate the flowerettes from the cauliflower stems. Cut the stems hasugiri and the heart sengiri. Save the outer leaves for soup.

Heat the oil and saute the onions, carrot, cauliflower heart and stem, cauliflower flowerettes and celery, in that order. Sprinkle on the salt and saute a few more minutes. Add boiling water and cook on a medium flame for 15 minutes.

Add the dissolved kuzu or arrowroot. When the liquid boils add the tamari soy sauce. When it boils again, serve it immediately.

Note: Do not overcook the cauliflower - it loses its shape and taste.

Variation: ⅓ cup seitan (87a.) can be added. Use 3 Tbsp. arrowroot flour to cover the seitan and allow it to sit for 5 minutes. Heat 1 Tbsp. of oil in a pan and fry the seitan 5 minutes on each side. Add the kuzu, tamari soy sauce and seitan at the same time.

Parsnip and Celery Nitsuke 48.

3 parsnips, cut in half moons ¼″
1 stalk celery, cut ¼″ hasugiri
1 tsp. sesame oil
⅓ cup boiling water

Saute the parsnips in a pressure cooker. After a few minutes add the celery and saute this a few more minutes. Add the boiling water and cover the pot.

Cook the nitsuke under pressure for 5 minutes. Before the pressure returns to normal, remove the vegetables and serve them hot.

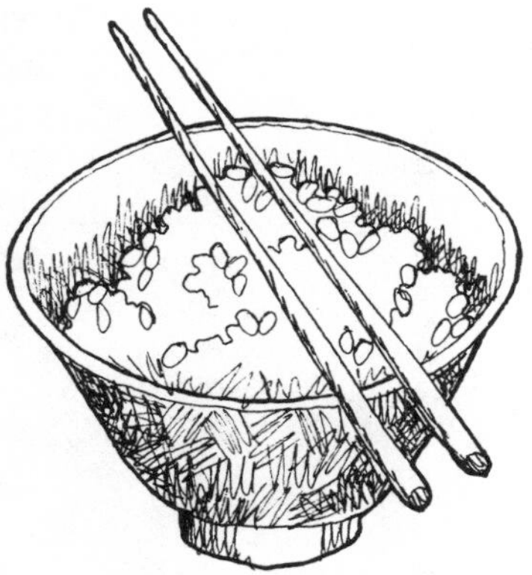

Rice Cream 49.

2 cups rice cream
5 cups boiling water
½ tsp. sea salt

Roast rice cream along with the salt in a dry pan. Stir frequently over a high flame until it is fragrant.

Place the pot in the sink and add 3 cups of boiling water to it. It will bubble slightly. After it stops bubbling, mix with a wooden spoon. Return the pot to the stove and bring the rice cream to a boil on a high flame. Add the rest of the boiling water, gently pressing around the inner edge of the pan so that the water seeps to the bottom. Do not stir the rice cream.

Cook covered on a medium flame using a hot pad for 30 minutes. Turn the flame to low and cook the rice cream another 30 minutes. Turn the heat off and serve the cereal after 5 minutes. If you plan to serve it later, keep it in the oven at 150°.

Rice Cream Powder

Prepared rice cream powder can be purchased in natural food stores and at macrobiotic outlets, but it is very easy to prepare at home and tastes much fresher. To make the powder, wash the rice and dry roast it (no oil) in a heavy skillet until it is golden in color and begins to pop. Grind it in an electric blender set at high speed or by hand in a grain mill.

Variation: Sweet rice cream powder is good mixed with regular. Make same as rice cream powder above. Use 1½ cups rice cream powder to ½ cup sweet brown rice powder, or try half and half. Determine your own proportions.

Millet with Chick Pea Sauce 50.

2 cups millet
2 med. onions, cut ¼″ mawashigiri
1 med. carrot, cut ¼″ sainome
2 pieces dried tofu, cut ¼″ sainome
2 cups chick peas (garbanzo beans)
5 cabbage leaves, cut into 1″ squares
1 Tbsp. sesame oil
1 heaping Tbsp. sesame butter
1 Tbsp. sea salt
1 heaping Tbsp. minced parsley

Wash and soak the chick peas 5 hours in 4 cups of water. Often there are stones or large pieces of dirt in them. Clean well. Pressure-cook the peas 45 minutes.

Wash and pressure-cook the millet in 4 cups of boiling water for 30 minutes and let sit.

Soak the dry tofu in warm water for 20 minutes until it has become soft. Rinse it in clear water, squeezing it each time until the water is clear. Cut as directed above.

Heat the oil and saute the onions until they are transparent, then add the dried tofu, cabbage and carrot. Add the cooked chick peas and enough boiling water to cover everything. Boil the sauce for 20 minutes. Add the salt and cook 20 minutes longer. Dissolve the sesame butter with some liquid from the chick peas and add to the pot, stirring slowly. Cook this 5 minutes more, then add tamari soy sauce to taste.

Open and stir the cooked millet. Mix from top to bottom and serve it with the chick pea sauce over it. Sprinkle the parsley on top for a garnish.

Hijiki with Lotus Root 51.

2 cups hijiki (sea weed)
4″ piece of lotus root, cut koguchigiri
1 Tbsp. tamari soy sauce
2 Tbsp. sesame oil
3 cups water

Wash the hijiki thoroughly to remove any grit. Cover it with water and let it soak for 15 minutes. Strain and reserve the water. Cut the hijiki into ½″ lengths.

Saute the lotus root for 10 minutes until it is sticky. Add the hijiki and saute another 5 - 10 minutes. Add the soaking water to cover the hijiki. After 30 minutes of boiling add the soy sauce and cook 30 minutes more. It should be a little salty.

If fresh lotus root is not available, dried lotus root that has been soaked can be used.

Variation: This recipe can be changed by adding burdock, carrots and onions.

Vegetable Ojiya 52.

3 cups cooked rice
7 cups vegetable soup (carrot, cabbage, onion, daikon)
3 Tbsp. barley miso *or*
2 Tbsp. tamari soy sauce

Bring the soup to a boil and add the rice. Cook this for 1 hour without stirring.

Add the miso or the soy sauce and bring the ojiya to a boil. Serve it immediately. When you are ready to serve this dish, stir it from top to bottom. Don't stir while it is cooking.

This is good on cold days to heat the body. See *Do of Cooking #4, Winter,* page 20, for variations on this recipe.

Clear Soup with Noodles *(Udon w/ Clear Broth)* 53.

1 8-oz. pkg. white noodles (udon)
2 heaping Tbsp. tempura crumbs (see 22c.)
5 scallions, cut thinly
1 sheet nori
8 cups boiling water
3 cups soup stock (see 16.)
½ tsp. sea salt
3 Tbsp. tamari soy sauce

Add the noodles to 8 cups of boiling water. When the liquid returns to a boil add 1 cup of cold water and bring to a boil again. Then turn off the flame and let the noodles sit a few minutes. Then stir them. To test if they are done, break one in half; it should be the same color throughout. If this is not so, they are not done and must be boiled again. When they are done, strain and wash the noodles a few times in cold water until they are completely cool. Then drain the excess water.

To 3 cups of soup stock add 2 cups of water and the salt and cook 20 minutes. Add tempura crumbs and bring the mixture to a boil. Add the tamari soy sauce and bring to a boil once again.

Place the noodles in bowls by the handful, using a twisting motion to separate each serving and make them attractive.

Serve these cold with hot soup stock over them. If the noodles are to be used hot, serve them immediately after boiling without rinsing.

Broccoli Nitsuke 54.

1 bunch broccoli
2 tsp. sesame oil
¼ tsp. sea salt
1 tsp. tamari soy sauce

Wash the broccoli and cut it in half, separating the flowers from the stem. Cut the stem from the cut end toward the bottom (don't cut the hardest part) in the ¼″ koguchigiri style. Separate the flowerettes into bite-size pieces. With the remaining hard stem, cut off the tough outer skin and cut core in ¼″ koguchigiri style. Throw the tough skin away.

Broccoli leaves can also be used — they are tender and delicious. After cutting, keep the stem parts separate from the flowerettes and leaves.

Heat the oil in a cast iron or stainless steel pan. Using a medium flame saute the stems and then the leaves, keeping the pan covered. Stir these occasionally and cook them until they become bright green in color. Then add the flowerettes. Stir occasionally until the color changes. Reduce to a low flame and sprinkle on the salt and tamari soy sauce. Stir the vegetables to distribute the salt evenly, and cook this for 20 minutes.

When the juice comes out of the vegetables and collects on the bottom of the pan, turn the flame to medium and cook the broccoli until it is tender. Do not stir the broccoli after it is tender — this will cause it to crumble. If you need to stir, pick up the pot and lightly toss the vegetables without using a spoon.

Cabbage Nitsuke 55.

1 small cabbage, cut in quarters
¼ tsp. sea salt
1 - 2 Tbsp. tamari soy sauce
2 tsp. sesame oil

After the cabbage is washed, remove the core and slice it thinly. Cut the leaves into 1″ squares.

Heat the oil and saute cabbage until it is bright green in color. Sprinkle on the salt and tamari soy sauce and stir the cabbage slowly. Cook it on a low flame covered for 5 minutes or until it appears watery. Turn the flame up to medium and cook until the cabbage is tender.

Turn off the flame and sprinkle on 1 tsp. of soy sauce. Stir and serve the cabbage immediately.

Variation: Add 1 heaping tsp. of miso dissolved in a small amount of hot water to the cabbage nitsuke. Bring it to a boil and serve.

Garlic Bread 56.

1 loaf French bread (see 58.), sliced in 1″ diagonal pieces
3 small cloves of garlic, grated
3 Tbsp. oil

Mix the oil with the garlic and let this sit for half a day. Brush both sides of each slice with this garlic oil and put all the bread together so that it looks like one loaf. Bake it in the oven at 450° for 45 minutes and serve it hot.

Carrot - Sesame Nitsuke 57.

2 large carrots, cut sengiri
2 Tbsp. white sesame seeds, washed and dried
2 tsp. sesame oil
½ tsp. sea salt
2 tsp. tamari soy sauce
⅓ cup water (if needed)

Heat the oil in a pan and saute the sesame seeds until they are slightly brown. Add the carrots and cover the pan. Cook this 5 minutes, stirring them occasionally. Add the salt and soy sauce and continue cooking covered on a low flame for 10 minutes.

When water comes from the vegetables, turn up the flame to medium and cook until tender. If no water comes, add the boiling water and cook the nitsuke about 10 minutes more.

Serve this dish warm.

French Bread 58.

4 cups unbleached white flour
3 cups whole wheat flour
2½ cups warm water
¼ tsp. dry yeast
1 Tbsp. sea salt
1 Tbsp. oil
bit of cornmeal

Add the yeast to warm water (105° - 115°) in a bowl.

When it is completely dissolved (about 5 minutes) add the oil and salt. Add the flour and make a dough. Knead for 20 minutes; the dough should be ear lobe consistency. Cover bowl with a wet cloth and let sit overnight until it has doubled in size.

If you are in a hurry, keep the dough on top of a gas stove for 4 - 5 hours until it has doubled its size.

Punch it down, divide it in half and shape it into loaves 4″ × 12″. Sprinkle a handful of cornmeal on a cookie sheet, place the loaves on the cookie sheet and gently rub them with cornmeal. Cover the bread with a wet cloth and let it rise about 1 hour or until it doubles in size.

With a sharp knife make 4 diagonal cuts ½″ deep in each loaf. Bake the bread at 450° for 45 minutes, or 350° for 1 hour.

Chinese Cabbage Pressed Salad 59.

1 whole Chinese cabbage, cut 1″ koguchigiri
1 - 2 tsp. sea salt

Mix the cut cabbage and the salt together. Press it in a Japanese salad press, or with a bowl and wooden cover with a heavy rock.

Let it sit a couple of days. When it tastes pickled or appetizing, it is ready to serve.

Vegetable Oden 60.

5 kombu rolls
5 cabbage rolls
5 stuffed age (64.)
1 medium carrot, cut 1″ hasugiri
5″ daikon, cut 1″ wagiri
5 small whole onions
7 cups soup stock (see 16.)
1 Tbsp. soy sauce
½ tsp. sea salt

Kombu rolls:
3″ × 15″ piece of kombu
2 med. burdock, cut in 3″ lengths, then 2 - 4 pieces lengthwise
2 med. carrots, cut in 3″ lengths, then 4 - 6 pieces lengthwise
kampyo (dried gourd strips)

Rinse the kampyo with warm water. Soak the kombu until it is soft. Strain kombu and allow to dry for 1 hour. Reserve soaking water for soup stock. Place the kombu on a cutting board. Place a piece of burdock and 2 pieces of carrot on the kombu and roll it twice. Cut the kombu and tie it with the kampyo.

Cabbage rolls:
5 large cabbage leaves
5 pieces of mock chicken (see 291.)
5 toothpicks

Cook the cabbage in salted boiling water until it is slightly soft. Remove and let cool. Place a piece of mock chicken in each cabbage leaf and fold it like a package. Secure it with a toothpick.

Stuffed age:
3 pieces age, rectangular shape (see 64.)
4-oz. pkg. of saifun (bean threads)
3 - 4 pieces of kampyo

Cut the age in half, place it in 2 cups boiling water and cook for a few minutes. Strain and let it cool. Place the saifun in boiling water for 2 minutes, then strain and cool it by rinsing in cold water. Slowly open up the age — it is like a bag. Pick up some of the saifun with your fingers, roll the long strands and stuff these inside the age. Tie the stuffed age with the kampyo. If there is extra saifun, roll it alone with your fingers and tie it with kampyo.

Place the kombu rolls on the bottom of a pan. Cover them with the soup stock, then add the daikon, onion, carrot, soy sauce and salt. Cook this for 2 hours. Then add the cabbage rolls, stuffed age and tied saifun and cook 20 minutes more.

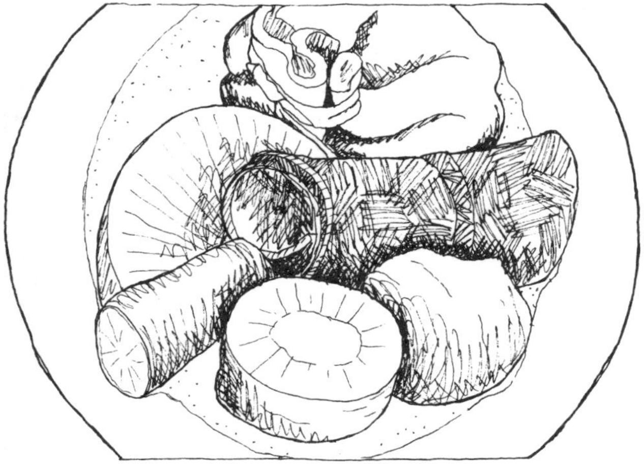

Serve each person a piece of each item and cover the serving with soup stock. Serve while it is hot. This is Vegetable Oden.

Oden Variation 60a.

2″ diameter, 10″ piece of daikon, cut 1″ wagiri
5 whole albi
2 small potatoes, cut into thirds
1 lb. whole string beans
1 carrot, cut ¼″ lengthwise
20″ piece of kombu
2 Tbsp. tamari soy sauce

Wash the kombu, saving the water. Let kombu dry a bit in a strainer; moist kombu is too slippery to roll.

Place a piece of carrot and 2 string beans in the kombu widthwise. Roll it twice, cut and secure it with a toothpick or kampyo (dried gourd strips).

Place the kombu rolls in a pot and cover with cold water. On top of kombu rolls place the daikon, albi, potato and soy sauce and bring to a boil. Cook it on a medium flame for 4 - 5 hours.

This dish improves as the vegetables cook and the flavors intermingle.

Green Pea Nitsuke 61.

2 cups whole dried green peas
4 cups water
1 tsp. sea salt

Soak the peas 5 - 6 hours after washing, and cook them under pressure for 45 minutes. Let the pressure come down, add the salt and cook the peas 20 minutes more.

Serve hot or warm.

Sakura Rice 62.

2 cups brown rice
1 Tbsp. tamari soy sauce
3 cups water

Cook same as 1a., using tamari soy sauce instead of salt. This sakura rice is very good with vegetable oden.

Variation: Add ¼ cup of sesame seeds.

Collard Green with Age Nitsuke 63.

1 bunch collard greens, cut 1″ koguchigiri
3 pieces of age, cut sengiri (see 64.)
2 tsp. sesame oil
¼ tsp. sea salt
1 Tbsp. tamari soy sauce

Wash the collard greens and cut. Saute them until they are bright green in color. Add the salt and soy sauce, cover the pan and cook the greens on a low flame for 5 minutes. Water will come out of the vegetables.

Turn the flame to medium. Add the age on top of the greens and steam for 5 minutes. Then mix the age into the vegetables and cook until they are tender (about 10 minutes).

Home-Made Age *(Deep-Fried Tofu)* 64.

1 block tofu, sliced into 8 pieces
Tempura oil - mixture of corn and safflower, equal proportions

Place a clean towel on a cutting board. On this place the tofu and cover it with another towel and cutting board to create pressure. Have the board slanted so the liquid will drain off. Let this sit for 1 hour.

Heat the oil and place the tofu strips in it, frying on high flame. Remove the tofu when both sides are golden in color. Serve it right away with grated daikon and tamari soy sauce.

Note: Tofu can be dusted with buckwheat flour or pastry flour 5 minutes before deep-frying. Age can also be pan-fried using less oil. This is good tasting.

Millet Croquettes 65.

1 cup millet
1½ cups boiling water
1 med. onion, minced
½ med. carrot, minced
½ block tofu, strained and pressed
3 Tbsp. oil
½ cup whole wheat pastry flour
1 tsp. sea salt
1 cup bechamel sauce (37.)

Place the washed millet in boiling water in a pressure cooker and cook it under pressure for 20 minutes. Turn off the flame and let the pressure come down to normal.

Saute the onion, carrot and tofu with 1Tbsp. oil and salt and cook these until they are tender. Add the warm millet and mix the vegetables and grain thoroughly. Let this cool to room temperature.

Add the flour, wet your fingers and shape the mixture into croquettes. Heat 2 Tbsp. of oil in a frying pan and cook croquettes for 7 minutes on one side, covered. Then turn and cook 5 minutes on the other side until they are golden brown.

Serve them with bechamel sauce and minced parsley.

Variation: Bulghur may be substituted for millet. Okara may be substituted for tofu.

Ohitashi *(Boiled Vegetables)* with Kiri-Goma 66.

7 stalks of Swiss chard (cut and separate stems from leaves)
1 handful of the outer leaves of lettuce
8 cups water
2 heaping tsp. sea salt

Bring the water to a boil and add the salt. Add the stems of the Swiss chard and cook them for 5 minutes on a high flame uncovered. Add the leaves of the Swiss chard and the lettuce. Cook these until the stems are tender.

Place the vegetables in a strainer with the leaves hanging over the edge, to quick-cool. If possible place near an open window. When the vegetables are cooled, squeeze off the excess water and cut them into 1½″ pieces. Sprinkle on soy sauce.

Serve them with kiri-goma (roasted and cut sesame seeds). Ohitashi can also be served with bonita flakes (dried fish condiment).

Burdock Carrot Roll 67.

2 med. burdock, cut into 5″ - 7″ lengths
2 medium carrots, cut same as above
1 cup whole wheat flour
3 tsp. sesame oil
¼ tsp. sea salt
4 tsp. tamari soy sauce
frying oil 3″ deep

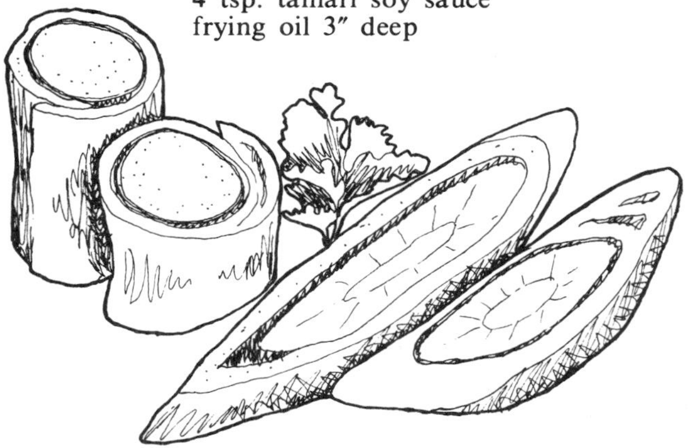

Saute the burdock in 1 tsp. oil. Add small amount of water and cook until they are half done. Add 2 tsp. soy sauce and cook until tender. Cool burdock.

Saute the carrot in 1 tsp. oil same as the burdock (use remaining tamari) and cool.

Add the salt and 1 tsp. oil to the flour and mix these thoroughly with your fingers. Add ⅓ cup of water and knead the dough lightly until it is slightly softer than ear lobe consistency. Roll out the dough to a ⅛″ thickness.

Roll the burdock in the dough, overlapping it about ½″ and seal it by pinching the ends of the dough closed. Prepare the carrot in a similar manner. Heat the oil and deep-fry the burdock rolls until the color of the dough changes. Turn the rolls over and fry them until both sides are brown. Remove them to a strainer and allow the excess oil to drain, then place them on a paper towel. Repeat this process for the carrot rolls.

Cut the burdock rolls into pieces 1½″ long and stand them on end. Cut the carrot rolls into pieces 1″ hasugiri. Serve with grated daikon.

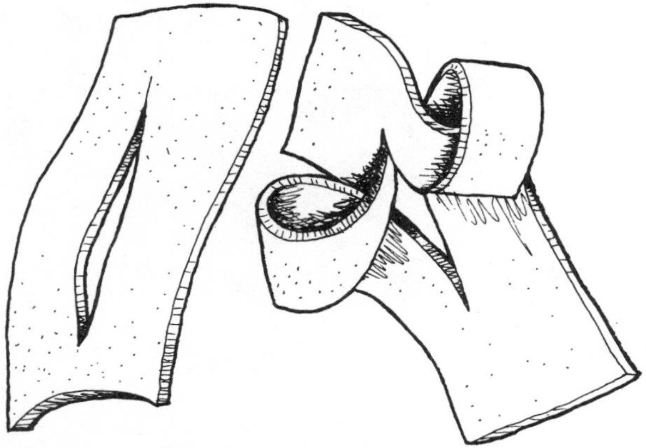

Karinto *(Deep-Fried Cookie)* 68.

1 cup leftover pie dough (see 31.)

Roll the dough out to ¼″ thickness and cut into rectangles 1″ × 5″.

Make a slit about 2″ long in the center of each rectangle. Take one end of the dough and pull it through this slit. It will resemble a piece of rope.

Deep fry it until it is crisp.

Split Pea and Macaroni Potage 69.

½ cup split peas
1 cup whole grain macaroni
2 med. onions, cut thin mawashigiri
½ med. carrot, cut ichogiri
½ stalk celery, cut ¼″ sainome
1 med. tomato, peeled and cut ¼″ sainome (optional)
2 tsp. sea salt
7 cups boiling water
1 tsp. sesame oil
tamari soy sauce to taste

Wash the split peas and soak them in 1 cup of water for 2 hours. Wash the macaroni and drain it.

Heat the oil and saute the onions until they are transparent. Add the tomato and saute it for 5 minutes with the celery and carrot. Saute each a few minutes.

Add the boiling water and split peas, including the soaking water. Bring the liquid to a boil and add macaroni and salt. Cook this 40 minutes or until it is tender. If necessary add more water. Add tamari soy sauce to your taste.

Sauteed Cabbage and Bean Sprouts 70.

½ head of cabbage, cut sengiri
2 cups bean sprouts
1 Tbsp. oil
½ tsp. sea salt

Cut the washed cabbage very thin. Wash the bean sprouts and drain them. Saute the sprouts on a high flame for a few minutes. When their color changes, put them in a bowl. Saute the cabbage on a high flame until the color changes slightly; then add salt and continue to cook cabbage until it is slightly soft.

Mix in the bean sprouts and serve hot. This is a crisp vegetable dish.

Azuki Winter Squash Nitsuke 71.

1 cup azuki beans
3 cups water
4 cups sliced winter squash (butternut, Hubbard)
½ tsp. salt

Soak the washed azuki beans in 1½ cups cold water at least 5 hours, or overnight. Bring them to a boil on a high flame, add ½ cup cold water and bring to a boil again. Repeat this procedure twice more and cook on low flame.

When the beans are tender (about 1 hour) add the sliced squash and salt and continue cooking until the squash is tender. Stir the nitsuke so that some of the squash gets mashed, similar to a puree.

This dish is beneficial to those who have diabetes or kidney diseases. It can also be used as a covering for mochi, or as filling for muffins.

Nori Kombu Nitsuke 72.

Kombu (leftover from soup stock), cut sengiri
1 pkg. nori, torn into 1″ squares
2 - 3 Tbsp. tamari soy sauce

Soak the nori in 1 cup of water. Cook the kombu in 1 cup of water until it is tender. Add the soaked nori and cook for 20 minutes.

Add soy sauce to taste and cook the nitsuke for 20 minutes more.

Home-Made Natto I 73.

5 cups soy beans
10 cups water
1 pkg. store-bought natto (4-oz.)
2 - 3 large porcelain or glass bowls with covers

Cook soy beans same as in 73a. After cooking, set soybeans aside to cool until 140°. Mix store-bought natto into the cooked soy beans.

During this process, keep the bowl warm (140°) by holding over hot water in another bowl or pan. Add mixed soy beans to the bowl until within 1½″ of top, and cover. Put the bowl in the oven with just the pilot light on (about 140°) and leave the beans overnight.

Then they should be ready to eat. After completely cooled, move natto to small containers. Natto can be stored frozen for a couple of months.

Home-Made Natto II

3 cups soy beans
6 cups water
Six 1-pint paper containers

Wash the soybeans and soak them in 6 cups of water overnight. Bring them to a boil on a high flame, then lower the flame and cook them 4 - 5 hours or until the beans are tender. Do not stir. Do not pressure-cook. Almost all the water will boil away; then strain.

Place 1 cup of the hot soy beans in each paper container and close them. Put all the filled containers in a double paper bag, tie it closed with string and put the bag in the oven. Leaving just the pilot light on (about 140°), keep the beans in the oven for 3 days and nights. They should then be ready to eat.

If you cook more beans, stack the containers on top of each other. Rotate the containers after the 2nd night and let them remain in the oven another full day.

Do not use your oven at all while you are making natto.

These fermented soybeans (natto) are very good for digestion and an excellent source of protein.

Uosoki

5 small fish, such as trout, sardines or smelt
⅓ cup pastry flour
½ lb. udon or whole wheat spaghetti
7 cups soup stock
5 small whole onions
3″ diameter center of Chinese cabbage, cut into 5 pieces, each 1″ thick
5 pieces of broccoli
5 pieces of cauliflower
5 string beans
2 tsp. sea salt
¼ cup tamari soy sauce
small bamboo skewers

Sprinkle the fish with 1 tsp. salt and 1 Tbsp. ginger juice and let sit for 1 hour. Cook broccoli, cauliflower and beans in salted water and place on bamboo skewers.

Cook the noodles until tender, then rinse and drain them.

Dust the fish with the flour, inside and out, and let sit 5 minutes. Deep-fry the fish in hot oil on a medium flame until they are golden brown on each side (about 20 minutes). The whole fish can be eaten.

Bring the soup stock to a boil, add 1 tsp. salt, ¼ cup soy sauce and the small onions. Cook the stock until the onions are half done, then add the Chinese cabbage. When the cabbage is soft, add the noodles and the fish and bring this to a boil. Add the vegetable kabobs, boil once more, and serve the uosuki hot.

This can be served from one dish at the table.

Variation: Tofu, mochi, croquettes, age or gluten cutlets can be substituted in this dish.

Northern White Beans with Miso 75.

2 cups Northern white beans
4 cups water
1 Tbsp. white miso (rice miso)
1 Tbsp. mugi miso (barley miso)

Wash the beans, soak them in water at least 5 hours and pressure-cook them for 30 minutes. After the pressure is down, remove the cover and add the two kinds of miso. Bring this to a boil and continue cooking on a low flame for at least 30 minutes.

You can also cook Northern white beans with white miso only.

Macaroni Salad 76.

1 cup white macaroni
⅓ cup green pepper, diced ¼″
2 red radishes, cut in half-moons
¼ cup coarse grated carrot
¼ cup celery, sliced thin
1 tsp. minced onion
½ tsp. minced celery leaf
½ tsp. sea salt
3 oz. mayonnaise (see 76a.)

Boil the macaroni in salted water until it is soft. Drain it and add 1 tsp. oil; sprinkle this over the top of the noodles and mix. Allow to cool.

Add the chopped vegetables, salt and mayonnaise and mix ingredients together thoroughly.

Mayonnaise Sauce *(Yield: 1 Cup)* 76a.

1 egg yolk
1 Tbsp. rice vinegar
1 tsp. sea salt
1 cup oil (corn, olive or sesame), boiled then cooled

Place the egg and salt into a glass bowl and beat them with a wisk. Add ½ tsp. of oil, drop by drop, while continually beating the mixture with a wisk. Repeat this process 2 - 3 times. After about 10 times, increase the oil to 1 or 2 Tbsp. until all the oil is used. Beat this along with the vinegar for a couple more minutes.

Your mayonnaise will turn out well if the egg yolk is very fresh. Thick oil is better than thin oil. In hot weather the mixing bowl and beater should be set in the refrigerator for a few minutes prior to using, to help thicken the ingredients.

If the oil separates, ½ a beaten egg white mixed into the mayonnaise may help. If you're not successful, make a new batch adding the old batch, instead of fresh oil, to the egg yolk.

More oil can be added if you desire thicker mayonnaise for decorating.

Mashed Potatoes 77.

10 lbs. potatoes
7 Tbsp. sesame oil
2 cups boiling water
3 cups milk
5 tsp. sea salt

Peel the potatoes and slice them into bite-size pieces. Saute them in sesame oil until they are transparent. Place them on a rack inside a pressure cooker with 2 cups of boiling water under the potatoes. Sprinkle on 2 tsp. of salt and cook for 20 minutes.

Let the pressure return to normal, remove the rack and mash the potatoes completely.

Add the milk and the remaining 3 tsp. salt and cook the mashed potatoes for 1 hour on a low flame.

Fried Chicken 78.

1 whole chicken, cut into pieces
3 cups pastry flour

Marinade:
2 Tbsp. tamari soy sauce
1 tsp. sea salt
2 heaping Tbsp. minced onion
1 Tbsp. sake
2 tsp. ginger juice

Mix the marinade and pour it over the cut chicken; stir occasionally and let sit for 1½ to 2 hours, so that all parts are equally seasoned.

Brush away the minced onion and dust the chicken with pastry flour. Let it sit for 10 minutes.

Heat 2 Tbsp. oil in a frying pan, place the chicken in pan and cover. Cook it on a medium high flame until it is slightly brown, about 5 minutes. Remove the cover, turn the chicken and cook without a cover on this side until it is slightly brown.

Place the chicken on a cookie sheet in a 250° oven for 1½ - 2 hours.

This way of preparing chicken using ginger, onion and sake which are yin, balances the yang of the chicken. The taste is especially good, and our experience is that we don't have bloody nightmares eating this dish as we sometimes do eating fowl prepared otherwise.

Gravy *(For Chicken)* 79.

Leftover oil
1 cup pastry flour
Cold water

Mix the oil from the cookie sheet (see previous recipe) and the leftover fry pan oil from the chicken.

Heat oil and saute 1 cup pastry flour until it is fragrant and is slightly brown in color. Let it cool and add cold water to make your gravy. You can also add the leftover marinade sauce and minced onions.

Home-Made Tofu and Nigari 80.

Tofu: 3 cups green soybeans
3 Tbsp. nigari or nigari powder (mix powder with 1 cup water)
6 cups water

Soak the washed soybeans overnight in water. In summer, 7 hours is long enough. In winter, if it is very cold, soak beans for 20 hours. To test the beans, cut one in half; the inside and outside of the bean should be the same color. Drain the beans, reserving the water.

Blend the beans in an electric blender or force them through a food mill, adding some of the soaking water, if necessary, to make a paste. Bring 10 cups of water to a boil and add the pureed beans immediately, to avoid spoiling. Bring beans to a boil without a cover and stir continuously. When the beans boil, sprinkle one cup of cold water on the beans to quiet the bubbling. Repeat this process 3 times, always bringing the water back to a boil.

Place cotton flour sacks in a wooden keg, pour the cooked bean mixture into a sack, and tie the sack. With the sack over the keg, squeeze it to remove most of the water. (This liquid - soy milk - is used to make the tofu.) Sprinkle the nigari over the surface of the water that has drained from the beans. *Note:* The bean water must be hot for the nigari to work. Let it rest 5 minutes. With a long-handled wooden spoon, make 2 deep strokes into the water at right angles to each other, as though to form a cross. Make these strokes slowly as though you were going to lift the bottom matter up to the top of the keg, dipping in at the sides of the keg and coming up again in the center. Let the mixture rest again for 10 minutes. Check to see if the liquid is separating. If not, sprinkle another tsp. of nigari over the water. Let stand 5 minutes and repeat 2 deep strokes with wooden spoon. Wait 5 minutes again.

You will see a white, thickened substance resembling scrambled eggs. Line a square slat-bottomed box with a clean cotton cloth and spoon out the thick white substance into it. Cover the top with a cloth and then a wooden lid. Place an empty quart jar on the lid for pressure, for 1 hour. Later increase pressure by using a ½ gallon jug containing 4 cups of water. About 1½ hours later, all water should be drained and the tofu is ready to use.

Place container in sink filled with water (plugged) and slowly remove cover and cloths in the water. Cover tofu with cold water for 30 minutes before serving. Cut into pieces 3″ × 4½″ and 1″ thick.

Note on tofu: The water should be squeezed from the tofu slowly, otherwise it becomes hard and breaks easily. If the water is light brown in color, do not use the tofu. Spring water is best to use when making tofu. Tofu will keep one week covered with water and refrigerated; change the water every 2 days to keep the tofu fresh. Tofu can best be served with any of the following: scallions, cut thin; bonita flakes; grated ginger. Tamari should be served in combination with any of the above.

Nigari: 5 lbs. crude gray sea salt
water
clean linen cloth

To make nigari, use damp sea salt. If the sea salt is dry, sprinkle it with some water until it is fairly damp.

Place the salt in the cloth and gather the sides to make a sack. Hang the sack in a cool, damp place to drain for several days. Collect the liquid that drips from the cloth sack in a pan or bucket.

This liquid is nigari.

Clear Soup with Tofu and Shingiku 80a.

3″ × 6″ piece of dashi kombu, cut in strips
⅓ cup chuba iriko (dried fish)
8 cups cold water
¼ block tofu, cut in bite-size pieces
5 shingiku tops
1 tsp. tamari soy sauce
½ tsp. sea salt

Add the kombu to 4 cups of water and bring to a boil on a medium flame. Add the chuba iriko and bring to a boil again, uncovered. Then strain and reserve this liquid. Add another 4 cups of water to the kombu and chuba iriko and bring this to a boil, covered. Cook 20 minutes, then strain it. Combine the liquids; this is the soup stock.

Use 3 cups of soup stock and 2 cups of boiling water for the clear soup. Add salt and cook it 20 minutes. Place the shingiku in a strainer and drop it into the boiling stock; remove it when it is slightly green. Keep the leaves where they can cool.

Add the tofu and soy sauce and bring the stock to a boil. Add the shingiku and serve it immediately.

Note: Watercress can be substituted for shingiku.

Tofu - Scallion Miso Soup 80b.

3 scallions, cut ¼″ koguchigiri
¼ block tofu, cut in ½″ cubes
3 Tbsp. barley or white rice miso
5 cups water

Dilute miso in ½ cup water.

Bring 5 cups water to a boil and add the scallion and tofu. Bring to a boil again, then reduce the heat until the stock is boiling slightly. Then add the softened miso.

Miso soup should not be boiled since the high temperature ruins the flavor and the nutrients. For this reason the miso is added last. After the miso has been added, the soup is ready to serve.

White Buns 81.

7 cups unbleached white flour
½ tsp. dry yeast
½ cup warm water
1 Tbsp. oil
1 Tbsp. sea salt

Dissolve the yeast in ½ cup warm water. After 5 minutes mix in 2 heaping Tbsp. of flour. Let sit in a warm place (top of the stove) for 10 minutes until the mixture bubbles.

In another bowl mix the remaining water, oil and salt with an egg beater. Place the flour in another bowl and add the yeast mixture. Use some of the oil/water mixture to get the yeast from the bowl, then add this mixture to the flour. Mix ingredients thoroughly with a wooden spoon, cover the bowl with a wet cloth and place in a warm spot until it doubles in size.

Wet your hands and punch the dough down. Turn it from top to bottom, cover again and let it rise a second time.

Sprinkle a 2″ high cake pan with corn meal, wet your fingers and shape buns 1″ in diameter and place them close together on the cake sheet.

Put them in a cold oven. Turn the thermostat to 450° and bake them for 1 hour, until their tops are slightly brown.

Variation: Sprinkle the tops with poppy or sesame seeds.

Amasake Cake with Cream Cheese Frosting *(3-layer)* 82.

5 cups whole wheat pastry flour
1 cup rolled oats
4 cups blended amasake (see 8.)
2 eggs, beaten
2 cups warm water
1 tsp. dry yeast
10 heaping Tbsp. whole wheat pastry flour
1 tsp. sea salt
6 Tbsp. corn oil

Frosting:
1 lb. cream cheese
2 Tbsp. honey
1 tsp. pure vanilla extract
⅓ cup raw milk

Dissolve the yeast in 2 cups warm water. Let it sit 5 minutes, add the 10 Tbsp. flour, make a batter and let sit for 5 minutes in a warm place.

Heat the amasake. While warm, mix with the yeast batter and add the eggs. Then add this to the 5 cups of flour using a wooden spoon to mix thoroughly.

Mix the oil, salt and oatmeal thoroughly with your hands. Mix with the batter, cover with a wet cloth and set in a warm place. It will double in size after 2 hours.

Punch down the dough with a wooden spoon and let sit another hour.

Oil 3 cake pans, dust them with a bit of pastry flour and pour in the batter. Even out with a spatula and bake at 350° for 45 minutes.

Frosting

Let the cream cheese soften at room temperature and slowly blend in the milk, honey and vanilla. Spread it between the layers, and as frosting on the cake. Create any design you wish.

Waffles 83.

4 cups whole wheat pastry flour
4½ cups water
2 cups cooked brown rice
1 cup cooked cereal
1 tsp. sea salt

Mix the rice with the water, then add the flour, salt and cereal. Blend these ingredients until you have a thick batter.

Heat a waffle iron and oil it. Ladle the batter into the hot iron and cook the waffles until they are crisp and brown (about 7 minutes).

Variation: Waffle batter can be used to make pancakes, which can be served with sliced apples or pears. In the winter, decrease the amount of pastry flour while substituting 1 cup or ½ cup of buckwheat flour. Mix the same as above.

Rice and Noodle Burger 84.

2 cups leftover fried rice (119.)
1 cup leftover noodles gratin (102.)
1 cup corn meal or bread crumbs
4 Tbsp. corn oil

Mix the flour, noodles and fried rice thoroughly. Wet your hands and make patties. Cover them with corn meal or bread crumbs and let them sit for 5 minutes.

Heat 2 Tbsp. of oil in a frying pan, place a layer of patties in the pan and cook them covered on a medium flame for 7 minutes. Turn them over and cook on the other side for 5 minutes or until both sides are golden brown.

Serve the 'burgers' hot with bechamel sauce (see 37.).

Chinese Cabbage, Onion, Carrot Nitsuke 85.

1 head Chinese cabbage, quartered and cored, then cut 1″ koguchigiri (strips)
2 onions, cut ¼″ mawashigiri
1 carrot, cut sasagaki
1 Tbsp. sesame oil
½ tsp. sea salt
1 - 2 Tbsp. tamari soy sauce

Heat the oil and saute the onions in a covered pan until they are transparent. Remove the cover and add the cabbage. Saute until it becomes bright green. Then add the carrot and saute the nitsuke a few minutes more. Sprinkle on the salt and soy sauce and mix the vegetables. Cover and cook them over a medium flame for 15 minutes or until they are tender.

Add tamari to taste, stir and serve.

Fresh Daikon Nitsuke 86.

1 daikon, cut sengiri
2 tsp. sesame oil
¼ tsp. sea salt
1 Tbsp. tamari soy sauce

Heat the oil and saute the daikon until it is transparent. Add the salt and soy sauce and cook the daikon on a low flame, covered, for 10 minutes.

When water comes from the daikon, turn the flame to medium and cook the daikon until it is tender.

Wheat Gluten 87.

10 cups whole wheat flour
4 cups unbleached white flour
5 cups cold water
2 tsp. sea salt

Mix the flours and add water in which the salt has been dissolved.

Knead the dough vigorously until softened. *Note:* This is best done by placing the bowl on the floor and working in a kneeling position. The dough will not make good gluten unless it is well-kneaded, so knead it for 20 minutes or longer. Set the kneaded dough in a bowl and leave it uncovered for 40 minutes.

Then add 8 - 10 cups of cold water and knead it vigorously. A cream-colored starch will appear from the dough. Change this water and repeat the process 5 - 6 times, reserving the starch-water for use in baking. Each time the water is changed it will become less sedimented. When there is only a slight bit of sediment in the water, stop the rinsing process.

Knead the dough until it becomes rubbery and place it in a strainer. About 5 cups of gluten dough will remain. In another pot bring 8 cups of water to a boil. Pull the gluten into thin 1″ pieces with your fingers and drop them into the boiling water. Boil the gluten until it rises to the top. Strain and reserve the water for use in cooking.

Wash the gluten in cold water until it is completely cold. Gluten must be completely cold before it is added to the soy sauce mixture when making seitan.

Gluten is easy to digest and is a good source of protein for sick people. It is eaten in all seasons, especially by vegetarians and those with a low intake of animal foods. Not only is it very important as a source of protein, it is also a very enjoyable food often used in sauces, stews, fried foods, etc.

Seitan is made from wheat gluten.

Seitan 87a.

1 Tbsp. sesame oil
1 Tbsp. minced ginger root
1 - 2 cups tamari soy sauce
5 cups cold cooked gluten (see 87.)

Heat the oil in a sauce pan and saute the minced ginger. Use fresh ginger only. Add the soy sauce, bring the mixture to a boil and drop in the pieces of gluten.

The amount of soy sauce used depends upon how long you intend to store the seitan. Use a larger amount of soy sauce for longer refrigeration.

Cook this covered on a low flame for 3 hours. Stir frequently.

Remove the cover and continue cooking until excess liquid is absorbed and evaporated.

Seitan is ideal as a seasoning in noodles au gratin, soups, stews, cooked with vegetables, etc. It will keep about 3 weeks in the refrigerator, and can be heated again.

Fresh Wheat Fu 87b.

- 5 cups wheat gluten, separated into 2 parts (87.)
- 8 cups water
- 3 cups whole wheat pastry flour
- 3 cups sweet brown rice flour

Knead one part of the wheat gluten with 3 cups of the mixed flours. Gluten is very sticky so kneading will be difficult at first. After about 20 minutes of kneading the dough will become smooth.

Repeat as above for the remaining gluten and flour mixture. Pat out each piece of floured gluten into a rectangle about 5″ × 6″ and 2″ thick.

Bring the water to a boil and drop in one rectangle. Once the water comes to a boil again, lower the flame and let it simmer for 20 minutes. Repeat for second rectangle. If using a steamer, steam the gluten pieces over a high flame for 30 minutes.

Remove the gluten with a ladle and place it on a platter to cool. Reserve the water to use in cooking or baking. Cut the gluten into strips ½″ wide. The reserved water and the cooked fu can be stored in the refrigerator for 1 week.

Fu can be used in a variety of vegetable dishes or deep-fried and served with noodles or stew.

Boiled Fu 87c.

- 3 cups soup stock (see 16.)
- 3 cups water
- Wheat fu, made from whole wheat pastry or sweet brown rice flour (see 87b.)
- 1 tsp. sea salt
- 3 Tbsp. tamari soy sauce

Bring the soup stock and water to a boil and add the soy sauce and salt. Drop in the wheat fu (cubed) and simmer it over a medium flame for 30 minutes. Wheat fu will expand in size during cooking.

Fried Fu *(Gluten Cutlet)* 87d.

- 1 cup whole wheat pastry flour
- 5 strips cooked fu (see 87b.)
- 2 cups tempura batter (see 22.)
- 2 cups corn meal or bread crumbs
- oil for deep-frying

Dust the strips of fu with pastry flour, then dip them into tempura batter. Cover each strip with corn meal and let sit on a plate for about 5 minutes.

Deep-fry them in hot oil (350°). Turn them after the strips rise to the top of the oil. Cutlets take about 5 minutes to cook. Remove them from the oil with a slotted spoon and place in a strainer set inside another pan to drain the excess oil. Serve.

Serving suggestions: Cut carrots and cabbage leaves into thin strips and saute them in a small amount of oil with a pinch of salt, over a high flame for about 5 minutes. Make a bed of the sauteed vegetables in the center of a serving dish and place the cutlets on top. Garnish this with red radishes cut into flower shapes.

Cutlet Kabobs 87e.

4 carrots
3 burdock roots
15 Brussels sprouts
1 tsp. sea salt
3 strips cooked fu (see 87c.)
2 cups tempura batter (22.)
2 cups corn meal or bread crumbs
12 - 15 bamboo or wooden skewers
1 cups pastry flour
tempura oil

Cut each piece of fu into 6 pieces. Cut the vegetables into 'logs' 1½″ long. Brussels sprouts are left whole.

Boil the carrots in just enough salted water to cover them for about 15 minutes. With the burdock, use only the upper portion (to maintain a diameter of about ¾″) and pressure-cook for 15 minutes with ½ tsp. salt and ½ cup of water. If you boil the burdock, cook it about 45 minutes in salted water. Cook the Brussels sprouts in 2 cups of salted water for 5 minutes uncovered, then drain and cool them.

Dip the vegetables first into the flour, then into the batter and finally into the corn meal or bread crumbs. Let them sit on a plate for 5 minutes. Deep-fry them in hot oil (350°) until golden in color. Follow the same procedure with all the pieces of wheat fu, and drain (as in 87d.).

Alternate pieces of wheat fu with vegetables on the skewers.

Serving suggestion: In the center of a platter, make a bed of string beans or snow peas that have been cooked in salted water. Surround them with a layer of salad greens, and arrange the Cutlet Kabobs on top of the leaves. For variation, please see 88.

Fried Saifun *(Dried Bean Threads)* 88.

1 2-oz. pkg. saifun (harusame)
1 head lettuce, cut ¼″ sengiri
1 lemon, cut into 6 pieces
oil

Heat the oil for deep-frying. Pick up 10 strands of dry saifun and place them in the oil. Stir quickly with a circular motion using chopsticks, making the noodles into spirals.

Make 6 spirals and then strain them until the excess oil is drained.

Serving suggestion: Make a bed of lettuce on a platter and place the spiraled saifun in the middle of the lettuce. On the sides of the noodles, arrange 2 Cutlet Kabobs (87e.) and 1 slice of lemon.

Daikon and Daikon Leaves Pressed Salad 89.

1 daikon, cut sengiri
Daikon leaves, cut very thin
1 Tbsp. sea salt

Place the daikon leaves in a suribachi or bowl, add 1 tsp. salt, stir and knead them for about 5 minutes. Green juice will come out of the vegetables. Squeeze out the excess water and throw away this green juice.

Mix the cut daikon with the leaves and the remaining salt thoroughly and press in a salad press overnight.

It is then ready to be served, after the juice over the vegetables has been removed.

Variation: 1 Tbsp. chopped shiso leaves mixed with ½ tsp. lemon juice can be added before pressing the salad.

This salad is a good balance for heavy foods.

Oatmeal Cookies 90.

1 cup whole wheat or pastry flour
½ cup uncooked rolled oats
½ tsp. sea salt
1 Tbsp. raisins, chopped
1 Tbsp. nuts (almonds or walnuts)
1½ Tbsp. sesame seeds
2 Tbsp. oil

Mix the oil and the flour so that the oil is distributed evenly throughout the flour. Add the remaining dry ingredients. Add enough water to form a sticky dough and drop it by the heaping teaspoonful onto a cookie sheet which has been lightly sprinkled with corn meal.

Bake the cookies at 450° for 30 minutes, or until they are slightly brown.

Saifun Nitsuke 91.

1 2-oz. pkg. saifun (bean threads)
3 med. onions, cut ¼″ mawashigiri
1 handful string beans, cut in
2″ pieces (optional)
1 carrot, cut sasagaki
½ head of cabbage, cut into 1″ squares
1 Tbsp. sesame oil
½ tsp. sea salt
2 Tbsp. tamari soy sauce

Place the saifun in boiling water, turn off the heat and let it soak for at least 5 hours. Drain, then cut in 2″ koguchigiri.

Heat the oil and saute the onions until they are transparent. Add the string beans and saute them, covered, until the color becomes bright green. Then add the cabbage and saute it until its color changes. Add carrots and saute a few minutes. Add salt and soy sauce and cook the vegetables on a low flame for 10 minutes.

After liquid comes out of the vegetables, cook them on a medium flame until they are tender. Add the saifun and stir well. Cook 10 minutes longer with a cover on the pot.

Add more salt or tamari soy sauce according to your taste.

Mustard Green and Carrot with Tempura 92.

1 bunch mustard greens, cut 1″ koguchigiri
1 med. carrot, cut sengiri
5 pieces of leftover tempura (see 22.)
¼ tsp. sea salt
1 tsp. sesame oil
1 Tbsp. tamari soy sauce

Saute the mustard greens until they are bright green in color. Add the carrots, saute a few minutes, then add the salt and the soy sauce. Cook this for 5 minutes on a low flame.

After water comes out of the vegetables, raise the flame to medium. Cook the vegetables until they are tender.

Add the tempura and mix it in with the vegetables. Cook the nitsuke until the tempura is warm and serve it.

Halvah 93.

4 cups whole wheat flour
14 cups water
½ cup currants
½ cup walnuts
4 apples, cut thin
2 tsp. cinnamon
2 tsp. sea salt

Dry-roast the flour until it has a nut-like fragrance. Remove it from the pan and let it cool.

Chop the walnuts.

When the flour cools, add 8 cups of cold water to it and mix thoroughly. Add 6 cups of boiling water, mix and bring all the ingredients to a boil. Add the currants, walnuts, apples and salt. Cook 1 hour on a low flame in a covered pot.

Add the cinnamon and cook 5 minutes more. Let it cool, then slice and serve it.

Muffins 94.

1 cup kidney beans
2 cups sliced yams or winter squash

Batter: 1 egg (optional)
4 cups water
4 cups whole wheat pastry flour
1 tsp. sea salt

Soak the washed beans in 3 cups of water for 5 hours.

Saute the yams (or squash), add the beans and pressure-cook this for 45 minutes. Let the pressure return to normal. Add ¼ tsp. salt and cook 20 minutes. Mash the mixture a few times. This is the filling.

Mix the egg with the water, flour and salt. It will become like a thick tempura batter.

Heat and oil the muffin pans; place them on the stove to warm them. Add 1 Tbsp. of batter, then 1 heaping tsp. of filling into each muffin section. Cover each with more batter. Bake the muffins at 450° for 45 minutes in the oven. Remove when they are golden brown.

Pan-Fried Fish 95.

5 pieces of flounder or other fish fillet
1 tsp. ginger juice
1 Tbsp. tamari soy sauce
1 Tbsp. water
2 Tbsp. oil

Marinate the fish in ginger, soy sauce and water for 20 minutes.

Dust the fish with pastry flour and let it sit for 10 minutes. The flour will absorb the excess liquid on the fish.

Heat 2 Tbsp. of oil in a frying pan. When the oil is hot, lower the flame to medium and place the fish in the pan. Cook it covered for 5 minutes. When the fish is slightly brown, turn it over and cook it on the other side until slightly brown also. Serve it hot.

Rice Kayu *(Soft Rice)* 96.

4 cups cooked brown rice
8 - 10 cups boiling water
¼ tsp. sea salt

Cover the rice with the boiling water and salt and cook it for 30 - 40 minutes in a pressure cooker under pressure. When you place it in the pressure cooker, don't stir it.

When the pressure returns to normal, mix the rice and serve it hot.

Scallion Miso 97.

1 bunch scallions, cut ¼″ koguchigiri
1 Tbsp. sesame oil
1 heaping Tbsp. mugi miso (barley miso)

After washing the scallions, cut and separate the roots from the stem. Cut the roots very thinly.

Heat the oil and saute the roots until they are slightly brown. Add the leaves (green parts of scallion) and saute them until their color changes slightly.

Spread the miso on top of the scallions and cover. Cook them for 5 minutes — the miso will soften. Stir it gently and saute until the miso has a fragrant smell.

Note: Scallion miso is good for the heart, for rheumatism, the brain and all yin diseases. It is a very good condiment with rice cream, rice kayu and cooked cereal.

Mustard Green Pressed Salad 98.

1 bunch mustard greens
1 tsp. sea salt

Wash the greens. Boil 8 cups of water and dip the greens in the boiling water using a high flame and no cover.

When their color changes, remove them and let them cool. Squeeze out the excess water. Cut the greens into 1″ pieces. Mix in the salt, place the greens in a salad press for one day, and serve them.

The taste is a little bit hot and good.

Wheat Cream 99.

2 cups wheat berries
8 cups cold water

Roast the wheat berries ½ cup at a time in a dry (not oiled) frying pan. Use a medium flame and roast until berries are dark brown in color.

Grind roasted berries into coarse (or fine, if you like) flour in a flour mill.

Roast this wheat powder until it is fragrant. Add 4 cups of water and mix together in a pot near the sink (not on top of the stove). Add the remaining water; try to get this additional water under the wheat cream batter.

Bring this to a boil on a medium flame, then lower the flame and cook covered for 1 hour. Turn heat off. After 5 minutes, mix thoroughly and serve hot.

Okara Nitsuke 100.

3 cups okara (soybeans which are leftover after making tofu)
1 cup burdock, cut sasagaki
1 cup carrot, cut sasagaki
1 cup onion, cut thin mawashigiri
1 tsp. sea salt
1 Tbsp. tamari soy sauce
2 Tbsp. sesame oil
½ cup scallion, cut ¼″ koguchigiri

Heat the oil and saute the burdock with cover on. After 5 minutes remove the cover and cook same as 2a. or 43. The burdock will smell sweet.

Remove the cover, add the onions and saute them until they are transparent. Add the carrot, saute it a few minutes, and sprinkle on the salt and soy sauce at the same time. Cover the pan and cook the vegetables until they are tender.

Put the okara on top of the vegetables, press it down and cook on a low flame covered for 30 minutes. The okara will get steam-cooked.

Stir the vegetables and the okara together thoroughly. Sprinkle with chopped scallions, stir again and serve immediately.

Sauteed Mustard Pickles 101.

2 cups old mustard pickles
1 Tbsp. sesame oil
¼ tsp. curry powder
1 - 2 tsp. tamari soy sauce

Heat the oil and saute the curry powder until it is brown.

Wash the old pickles, squeeze the excess water from them and place them in the pan with the curry. Saute this on a high flame for a few minutes.

Add the soy sauce to taste.

Buckwheat Noodles Gratin with Kuzu Sauce 102.

4 cups cooked buckwheat noodles
2 med. onions, cut mawashigiri
½ head small cauliflower, broken into flowerettes
½ stalk celery, cut hasugiri
1 carrot, cut sengiri
1 Tbsp. sesame oil
5 cups boiling water
2 heaping Tbsp. arrowroot flour or kuzu, diluted in 6 Tbsp. water
1 tsp. sea salt
2 Tbsp. tamari soy sauce

Saute the onions until they are transparent. Add the carrot and saute it a few minutes. Then add the celery, boiling water, cauliflower and salt and cook these for 20 minutes.

Add the dissolved kuzu and stir until it boils and thickens the mixture. Add the soy sauce to taste.

Place the cooked noodles in a glass baking dish and pour the sauce over them. Bake in a 450° oven until the sauce bubbles — about 40 minutes. Serve hot.

Vegetables with Tahini Sauce 103.

1 Tbsp. tahini or sesame butter
3 Tbsp. tamari soy sauce
2 stalks broccoli
1 small cauliflower
2 med. carrots

Boil each vegetable whole in salted water separately in this order: cauliflower, broccoli and carrot. Remove and let it cool, then slice cauliflower and broccoli into flowerettes. Cut carrot into bite-size pieces (rangiri).

Combine the tahini (or sesame butter) with the soy sauce and mix this with the vegetables. Serve.

Boiled Fresh Daikon with Lemon Sauce 104.

10 pieces of daikon, sliced 1″ thick wagiri
1 Tbsp. sweet brown rice
4 cups water

Place the sweet brown rice in a cotton bag. Tie it securely. Place it in the water with the daikon and boil them together. Cook this about 30 minutes, until the daikon is soft. Remove the daikon from the water and serve it immediately with the sauce.

Lemon sauce: 1 Tbsp. sesame oil
3 heaping Tbsp. barley miso
½ cup boiling water
½ tsp. lemon rind
2 Tbsp. lemon juice

Saute the miso in oil until it is fragrant. Add the boiling water, bring to a boil, then turn off the heat. Mix in the lemon rind and let it cool. Mix in the lemon juice, and serve it over the daikon.

This sauce is good for digestion, especially with any fried foods.

Baked Smelt 105.

10 smelt
1 Tbsp. ginger juice
3 tsp. sea salt

Clean the fish and sprinkle it with the ginger juice and 2 tsp. of sea salt. Let it sit for 30 minutes.

Oil a cookie sheet and place the fish on it. With your fingers about 12" above the fish, sprinkle 1 tsp. of salt over the fish. As it bakes it will form a nice white glaze.

Bake it at 450° for 45 minutes and serve it hot.

Buckwheat Noodle Burger 106.

2 cups cooked buckwheat noodles, or left-over Noodle Gratin (102.)
1 cup okara (80.) or 1 cup any cooked cereal
½ cup whole wheat pastry flour
leftover ginger from making ginger juice, or ½ tsp. grated ginger
1 tsp. sea salt

Mix all the above ingredients, adding a little water as needed. Make patties and fry them in an oiled pan for about 7 minutes on each side.

Serve them hot.

Sauteed Carrot with Kidney Beans 107.

2 cups kidney beans
4 cups water
2 cups carrot, cut ¼" sainome (diced)
1 tsp. sesame oil
2 Tbsp. miso *or* 1 tsp. sea salt

Soak the kidney beans overnight after washing them.

Saute the carrots for 5 minutes. Add the soaked beans and cook this under pressure for 45 minutes. Let the pressure return to normal.

Add the miso or salt and cook the dish 20 minutes longer.

Squash Bread-Cake 108.

5 cups pureed squash
8 cups whole wheat flour
3 tsp. sea salt
1 Tbsp. cinnamon
1 cup currants
1 cup chopped walnuts

Cook the cut-up squash in a pressure cooker with 1 tsp. salt and 1 cup boiling water for 10 minutes under pressure. Puree this, add the currants and cool the mixture.

Mix the remaining ingredients thoroughly, add to the puree and let it sit for 3 hours.

Oil 2 small bread pans and place the dough in the pans (after dividing dough in half). It will be a wet dough.

Wet your finger and spread the dough out. Bake it for 1½ hours at 350°. Do not pre-heat the oven.

Gomashio 109.

10 Tbsp. whole sesame seeds
1 Tbsp. sea salt

Fill a bowl with cold water, add the sesame seeds to it and stir until half the seeds float on top of the water.

Pour this into a fine mesh strainer. Add more cold water to those sesame seeds remaining in the bowl, stir and strain them again. Repeat this until all the seeds are washed and strained and only sand and dirt remain on the bottom of the washing bowl. Let the seeds drain in the strainer for 30 minutes, placing a sponge or towel underneath the strainer to catch the excess water. If you have the time, let them drain ½ a day.

Heat a cast-iron frying pan and roast the salt, stirring constantly until the acid smell is gone. Place this roasted salt in a suribachi and grind it very finely.

Roast the sesame seeds using a medium flame. Stir them constantly until all the seeds are browned equally. When the roasted seeds crush easily they are done. Taste a few — if they taste good they are done.

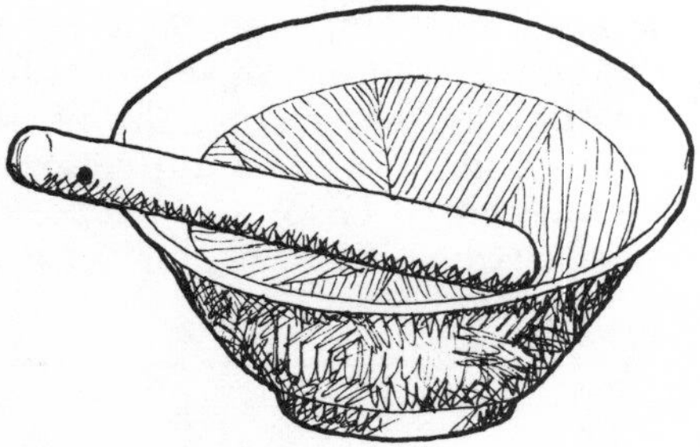

Add the roasted seeds to the ground salt in the suribachi. Grind the roasted salt and seeds together gently and evenly until ⅔ of the seeds are crushed. Don't grind too forcefully.

Cool the gomashio completely and place it in a glass or porcelain jar that has a cover. Keep it tightly covered when you are not using it.

Vegetable Stew 110.

5 onions - 2 minced, 3 cut ¼″ mawashigiri
3 small turnips, cut ¼″ mawashigiri
1 carrot, cut rangiri
2 Tbsp. sesame oil
⅔ cup whole wheat pastry flour
1 Tbsp. sea salt
1 heaping Tbsp. minced parsley
1 tsp. grated ginger
7 cups boiling water

Heat up 1 Tbsp. oil and saute the flour until it is fragrant. Set it aside to cool.

Heat the other Tbsp. of oil and saute the minced onions on a medium flame until they are brown. Add the other cut onions and saute until transparent. Add the turnips, saute a few minutes and then add the carrot. Saute these a few minutes more, add boiling water and salt and cook the stew for 30 minutes.

Make a paste from the roasted flour and some of the cooking liquid. Add this to the vegetables and boil 10 minutes on a low flame.

Add the ginger and boil it again. Serve it immediately, garnished with parsley.

Chick Pea Spread 111.

2 cups cooked chick peas (garbanzo beans)
1 tsp. sesame oil
3 small cloves of garlic, grated
1 heaping Tbsp. sesame butter
½ tsp. sea salt

Blend the cooked chick peas with some water reserved from their cooking (see 17.).

Heat the oil and saute the garlic until it is brown in color. Add the blended chick peas and the salt. Bring this to a boil and cook on a low flame for 20 minutes.

Dilute the sesame butter with some liquid from the cooking chick peas and add this to the chick peas. Bring this to a boil once more.

Let cool, add a bit of lemon juice, mix well and serve.

Deep-Fried Fish with Kuzu Sauce 112.

2 lb. perch, whole
½ cup arrowroot flour

Marinade: 1 Tbsp. sake
2 Tbsp. tamari soy sauce

Clean the fish with a paper towel to take up the excess water. Cut it in 3 places on a deep diagonal until you reach the bone. Do this on both sides. Marinate it for 1 to 2 hours.

Using the arrowroot flour, dust the fish inside and out and let it sit for 20 minutes.

Heat the oil for deep-frying. When the oil is hot enough, turn off the heat for 5 minutes and let it cool a bit. Then add the fish and cook it on one side for 30 minutes using a medium flame. (If the fish is too big for the pan, spoon hot oil over the parts which are not in the oil.) Turn the fish over and cook it on the other side for 20 minutes more.

Place it in a strainer to drain the excess oil. Immediately cover with hot kuzu sauce and serve it.

Kuzu Sauce: 1 block tofu, cut into 1″ squares (see 80.)
7 fresh mushrooms, cut into 8 pieces each
3 shiitake mushrooms, soaked in warm water, cut into ¼″ strips
2 green peppers, cut into 1″ squares
2 Tbsp. arrowroot, dissolved in ¼ cup cold water
2 cups water (from soaking shiitake mushrooms)
1 Tbsp. sesame oil
2 Tbsp. tamari
1 tsp. sea salt

Heat the oil on a high flame and saute the green pepper, fresh mushrooms and the shiitake mushrooms for a few minutes. Add the soaking water from the mushrooms along with 1 tsp. salt and cook for 5 minutes without a cover. Add the tofu and 2 Tbsp. soy sauce with the dissolved arrowroot. Bring this to a boil, let it thicken and serve it hot over the fish.

Egg Foo Yung 113.

6 eggs, beaten
1½ cups minced onion
2 cups bean sprouts
1½ tsp. sea salt
3 Tbsp. sake
2 Tbsp. oil

Heat 1 Tbsp. of oil and saute the onions until they are transparent. Add ¼ tsp. salt, then remove to a bowl to cool.

Heat the other Tbsp. of oil, saute the bean sprouts on a high flame and add ¼ tsp. salt. Cook a few minutes. Remove them to another bowl to cool.

Beat the eggs, add 1 tsp. salt and all of the sake. Mix. Add the cooled vegetables and mix thoroughly.

Oil a frying pan, scoop out the mixture with a ladle and place about 3 small pancake-sized omelettes in the pan. When they are half done, turn over and cook them on the other side until browned. Cover with egg foo yung sauce.

Sauce: ¼ cup fresh green peas
5 med. shiitake mushrooms, soaked in 1 cup warm water and each cut in 8 pieces
1 Tbsp. oil
½ tsp. sea salt
1 Tbsp. arrowroot flour
2 Tbsp. tamari soy sauce

Heat the oil and saute the mushrooms. Add the peas and saute them until they become bright green. In a separate pan, boil the water from soaking the mushrooms. Add this to the vegetables with the salt and cook 5 minutes without a cover.

Add the tamari soy sauce and the dissolved arrowroot and cook until it is thick. This is the sauce for the egg foo yung. Cover egg foo yung with the hot sauce and serve it immediately.

Saifun Salad with Mayonnaise Dressing 114.

2 oz. saifun (bean threads)
¼ head cabbage, cut in 1″ pieces (core removed)
1 med. carrot, cut thin hasugiri
1 med. cucumber
1 peach, 1 apple, cut into 8 pieces each, sliced ¼″ thick fan shape (optional)
8 cups water
2 heaping tsp. sea salt

Boil 3 cups of water, add the saifun and cook it for 5 minutes. Strain it and set it aside to cool.

Cook the cabbage in remaining water with salt. Bring it to a boil in an uncovered pot. Cook until slightly tender, then set it aside to cool.

Cook the carrot in the remaining water until it is slightly tender. Strain and set aside to cool. The remainder of the water can be reserved for clear soup.

Cut about ½″ off the stem part of the cucumber and rub it with salt. This will remove some of the bitterness. Cut it in half lengthwise, then cut it thinly in fan shapes. Place in a salad press, sprinkle with ½ tsp. salt, and press for 10 minutes. Form into fan shape by pushing down the cut edges.

Dressing: 1 egg, beaten
2 tsp. sea salt
½ cup oil
3 Tbsp. orange juice
1 Tbsp. lemon juice

Add the 2 tsp. salt to the beaten egg and continue beating as you add the oil by drops (using a chopstick) until one third of the oil is used. Add a further third of the oil by using a tsp., and the remaining third by Tbsp. Continue beating until it is creamy. When it becomes thick, add the lemon juice and the orange juice. Add the minced onion and let this sit for 20 minutes.

Cut the cold saifun in 2″ lengths. When all the vegetables are completely cooled, mix with the fruit and the mayonnaise dressing. Use fan-shaped (suehiro) cucumbers to decorate, opened so that their point is away from the center.

Egg Drop Soup 115.

1 small egg, beaten
3 scallions, cut ¼″ koguchigiri
¾″ piece of dashi kombu, cut in comb shape
7 cups of cold water
½ tsp. sea salt
2 tsp. tamari soy sauce

Soak the kombu for 5 hours, then boil it for 20 minutes.

Remove the kombu from the water, add the scallions and boil them on a high flame without a cover. Add the salt and the soy sauce. Pour the egg using your left hand, and with your right hand stir the broth so that the egg remains separated.

After the egg has cooked, shut off the heat and serve the soup immediately.

Egg Drop Soup *(Variation)* 115a.

1 med. onion, cut thin mawashigiri
1 heaping Tbsp. scallions, cut ¼″ koguchigiri
1 heaping Tbsp. chirimen iriko
1 egg white
1 tsp. sesame oil
5 cups water
¼ tsp. sea salt
1½ tsp. soy sauce

Saute the onion in oil. Add the chirimen iriko and saute until the fish smell is gone. Add the water and salt and cook this for 20 minutes.

Add the soy sauce. Beat the egg white and pour it into the soup. Be careful to stir the soup constantly as you pour, so that the egg cooks in small pieces.

Add the scallions, boil and serve the soup hot.

Tuna Sashimi 116.

1 lb. fresh tuna fillet
1 5″ size daikon
1 piece of ginger, grated
3 - 4 Tbsp. tamari soy sauce

Slice the tuna so it is in pieces 1″ thick. Then cut it into ¼″ × 2 - 3″ pieces.

Layer it on a serving dish and serve it cold. Serve with fresh raw daikon cut into thin matchsticks. Soak the daikon in ice water for 10 minutes to make it crisp.

Serve grated ginger or grated horseradish on the side as a condiment.

Pineapple and Apple Open-Face Pie 117.

1 pineapple, peeled and cut into ½″ strips
10 apples, each cut into 8 pieces and then into strips
1 cup apple juice
3 Tbsp. arrowroot flour, diluted in 6 Tbsp. cold water
1 tsp. sea salt

Pie Crust: 3 cups whole wheat pastry flour
3 Tbsp. oil
½ tsp. sea salt
1 cup cold water

Slice the pineapple, place on a cookie sheet and bake it in a 350° oven for 30 minutes or until it is slightly tender and lightly browned. Remove from the oven and let it cool. Then cut it into ¼″ cubes.

Slice the apples and cook them 10 minutes covered with apple juice. Cool them and mix them together with the pineapple and the diluted arrowroot.

Mix the oil, flour and salt. Rub the flour through your fingers until it has been saturated by all the oil. Add the cup of cold water and mix the dough with a fork. Do not knead it. Roll it out thinly and cover a pie pan with it.

Bake it at 350° for 10 minutes or until it is light brown. Remove from the oven and cool. (This recipe will make two pie shells.) Fill the pie shell generously with the cold pineapple filling and bake it at 350° for 30 minutes or until it is slightly brown and spotted.

Baked Squash with Sesame Sauce 118.

1 winter squash, cut in quarters

Sesame sauce: 2 Tbsp. sesame butter or tahini
6 Tbsp. tamari soy sauce
9 Tbsp. water

Place the squash on a cookie sheet and bake it in a 400° oven for 1 hour. Use a bamboo skewer to see if the squash is tender.

For the sesame sauce, mix all sauce ingredients and bring them to a boil. Serve the sauce over the squash.

Fried Rice 119.

7 cups cooked rice (see 1b.)
1 med. onion, cut thin mawashigiri
5 cabbage leaves, cut thin sengiri
1 stalk of celery, cut thin hasugiri
1 Tbsp. oil
½ tsp. sea salt
1 Tbsp. tamari soy sauce
1 Tbsp. minced parsley (mijingiri)

Heat the oil in a heavy iron pan and saute the onions until they are transparent. Add the cabbage and celery and saute them for 10 minutes.

Spread the vegetables over the bottom of the pan. Then put the rice on top of the vegetables and cover the pan. Do not stir. Cook on low flame. When steam rises from the rice, mix the rice and vegetables.

Cook them with a cover for 5 minutes until the rice is nice and hot. Shut off the heat and sprinkle on the soy sauce. Serve the dish immediately, garnished with parsley.

Note: If the rice is very dry, pour ½ cup boiling water around the edge of the pan. This will soften the rice.

Wild Pigeon, Fowl or Fish Shish-Kebab 120.

10 pieces of pigeon, fowl or fish, bite-size
2 onions, cut ¼″ mawashigiri
2 green peppers, cut ¼″ mawashigiri
10 scallions, cut 2″ koguchigiri
2 potatoes, pressure-cooked whole for 20 minutes, then cut into bite-size pieces, rangiri
2 Tbsp. sesame oil

Marinade Sauce: See 78.

Barbecue Sauce: Mix the following together:
½ cup tamari soy sauce
½ cup sake or sherry
2 Tbsp. ginger juice

Cover the fowl or fish with marinade sauce for 1 hour.

Skewer the onion, green pepper, scallion, potato and fowl. Heat a frying pan, add the 2 Tbsp. of oil and place all the kebabs in the pan. Cover and cook them 7 minutes on a medium flame. Turn each one over and cook 7 minutes on the other side. The onion will become transparent and the scallion will be bright green.

When they are done, dip the kebabs in the barbecue sauce and serve them immediately. If you have to wait, put them in the oven and cover them with a pie plate.

White Rice 121.

3 cups white rice
4 cups cold water

Wash the rice several times by firmly kneading it until the water turns white. Strain it and repeat washing it until the water is clear. Then drain it thoroughly.

Using a cast iron dutch oven or any heavy cooking pan, add the water to the white rice and cook it on a high flame, covered. After about 15 minutes steam will come from the side of the cover. Turn the flame to low and cook rice 15 minutes. Turn it off and let sit for 15 minutes. Then remove cover, mix rice from top to bottom, and serve.

Never take the cover off when cooking white rice.

If you ever become tired of eating brown rice, white rice is a pleasant change.

Tempura Sauce with Ginger 122.

½ cup soup stock (see 16. or 80a.)
½ cup water
2 - 3 Tbsp. tamari soy sauce
1 tsp. ginger juice

Bring the soup stock and the water to a boil. Add the soy sauce and turn off the heat. Take the pan off the stove, add the ginger juice and serve the sauce when it cools.

Ginger juice is made by grating a fresh piece of ginger. Take the grated ginger and squeeze it in your hand or through a clean kitchen towel. The leftover pulp may be used for Nuka Pickles mixture, or used for additional flavoring.

Chinese Cabbage Roll 123.

5 large Chinese cabbage leaves
1 bunch spinach
1 sheet nori sea weed
8 cups boiling water
1 heaping tsp. sea salt

Add the salt to the boiling water and place the cabbage leaves into the water with the leafy part up. Cook them uncovered. When the liquid boils, turn the leaves with chopsticks. Remove them when they are soft and set them aside in a strainer to drain and cool.

Add the spinach to the same boiling water and cook in the same manner as the cabbage. When it is done, place the leaves around the edge of the strainer to cool quickly.

Squeeze the Chinese cabbage leaves and the spinach separately on a sushi mat. Then place the sushi mat down and place the cabbage leaves flatly on it. Alternate the leaves until they cover the mat. Then place the spinach on top. Cover all but 1″ of the cabbage on each end.

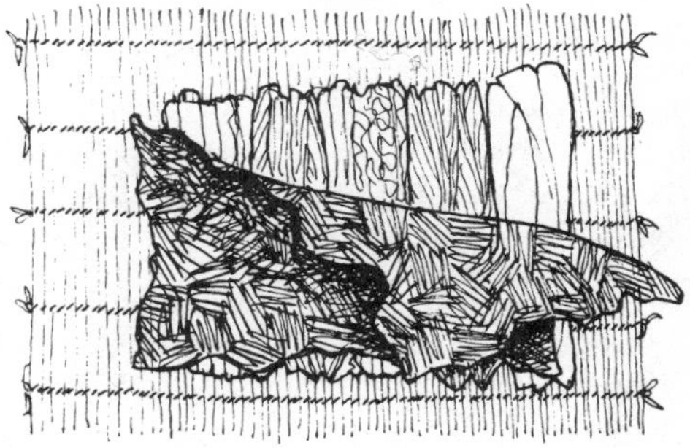

Place a sheet of nori on top of the spinach. Roll the mat and squeeze out any excess water. Cut the roll into 1″ pieces.

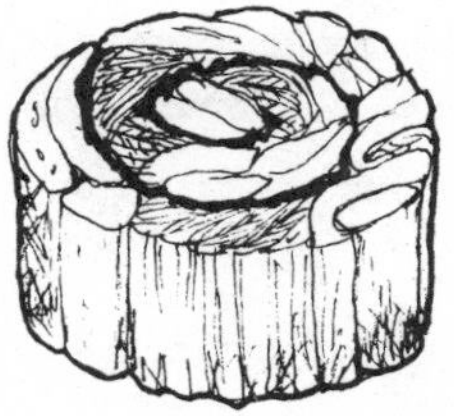

This dish is so colorful and tasty!

Apple Crisp 124.

4 cups sliced apples
1/3 cup whole wheat flour
1 cup uncooked rolled oats
1/2 tsp. sea salt
1 tsp. cinnamon
1 tsp. grated lemon rind
1/2 cup oil
1/8 cup water

Mix the oil and water together. Combine the rolled oats, flour and salt and mix this with the oil and water mixture. Be sure to mix all this together thoroughly with a fork. It should be somewhat moist.

Oil a baking dish and place the sliced apples in it, pressing them down with your hands so they are squeezed down a little. They will shrink as they cook. Sprinkle them with the lemon rind.

Place the flour mixture on top of the apples and bake them at 350° for 30 minutes or until all the apples are soft.

Variation: Place 1/2 cup of apple juice on the bottom of the pan and cut the apples larger. Or, you can double this recipe and make a 2-layer apple crisp.

Rice Balls 125.

3 cups cooked rice - for 8 rice balls
2 sheets of nori - cut each sheet into 9 pieces
Shio kombu
Umeboshi (salt plums)
Sea salt
Bancha tea, or cold boiled water

Hot or warm rice is best for making rice balls. Fill a small rice bowl with rice; this is a good way to measure the correct amount to use. Don't squeeze rice balls too hard when you shape them. Use your shoulder muscles instead of squeezing with your fingers. Your fingers should just shape the rice. The rice should be firm on the outside and soft in the center.

Before making rice balls your hands should be clean. If you wash with soap, make sure you completely rinse your hands to avoid soapy-tasting rice balls.

Put bancha tea in a bowl. Wet your hands in the tea and hold the rice in your left hand. In the center put 2 - 3 pieces shio kombu (see 126.) or a piece of umeboshi for flavor. The salt plum will also keep the rice from spoiling.

A pinch of salt to cover the rice ball will keep it moist and avoid drying. Cover rice balls with gomashio, shiso-goma, pickled shiso leaves or untoasted nori. Cut 9 pieces from one sheet of nori. (Fold in half lengthwise, then cut lengthwise so that you have thirds. Then cut widthwise into thirds, leaving nine pieces.) Cover each side of the rice ball with one piece. Nori is yin sea weed so not too much should be eaten at one time.

Don't wet your hand too much with tea or the rice will get soggy and spoil easily.

Rice balls are good for picnics and travelling. Cold rice doesn't usually taste good, but when made into rice balls it is more pleasant. Sometimes pregnant women find it difficult to eat brown rice, but they can usually eat it in the form of rice balls because a rice ball compresses the rice and makes it more yang. They become filled with the Ki or the life-energy of the person making them.

George Ohsawa used to cure sick people by serving them rice balls. One rice ball was cut in ten pieces and each piece was chewed 100 to 200 times. This helped sick people recover quickly. When you try to cure sick people, however, you must feel a deep and sincere desire that the sick person should get better. Your feelings are transmitted through the rice.

Shio Kombu 126.

8 oz. of dashi kombu
1 pint of tamari soy sauce

Cut the kombu into ½″ squares with a pair of scissors. Soak this overnight, covered with soy sauce.

Bring it to a boil over a high flame, then lower the flame and cook it 3 hours. Stir it occasionally. Kombu has natural sea salt which goes to the bottom of the pan. This will burn if not stirred occasionally.

Keep the kombu in a glass jar at room temperature. It can be kept a long time. Shio kombu is very good for fatigue: Put 2 - 3 pieces in a cup, add hot bancha tea and drink this brew. It is very refreshing. Shio kombu is also good inside of rice balls.

Note: If you use nishime kombu you must remove sand from the kombu. Use a wet towel to completely wipe the kombu, then cut and dry it for ½ a day on a sheet of paper until it is completely dry.

Squash Potage with Croutons 127.

1 med. acorn squash or any winter squash
2 med. onions, minced
1 Tbsp. sea salt
1 Tbsp. sesame oil
3 Tbsp. whole wheat pastry flour, roasted
1 tsp. tamari soy sauce
1 Tbsp. minced parsley
½ cup sliced bread or corn chips (see 58.)

Saute the onions in a pressure cooker, then add the squash which has been cut into small pieces. Saute these vegetables a few minutes, add the salt and enough water to cover. Bring it up to pressure on a high flame, then turn down flame and let the vegetables cook 20 minutes under pressure. Shut off the flame and allow pressure to return to normal.

With a Foley food mill, puree the vegetables.

In a separate bowl add water to the flour and make a thin batter. Add this to the squash mixture. Cook it 20 minutes and add soy sauce to taste.

Garnish with parsley and bread croutons or corn chips.

Bread Croutons

Cut 2 pieces of yeasted bread into ½″ cubes. Heat oil and add the cut bread. Cook over a medium flame and turn the croutons until all sides are golden brown. Strain and reserve the excess oil. Let croutons cool before using.

Pan-Fried Gyoza with Lemon Sauce 128.

Crust: 1 cup whole wheat flour
1 cup unbleached white flour
¾ cup boiling water
1 tsp. sesame oil
1 tsp. salt

Filling: ¼ cup minced onion
¼ cup scallion or chives, minced
½ cup Chinese cabbage, minced
½ cup cabbage, minced
1 tsp. ginger juice (grate, squeeze ginger and discard remains)
½ tsp. sea salt
1 tsp. tamari soy sauce
1 tsp. sesame oil
1 heaping Tbsp. minced seitan or chicken
2 heaping Tbsp. fresh bread, cut in ¼″ squares

Lemon sauce: 1 Tbsp. lemon juice
3 Tbsp. tamari soy sauce

Add the boiling water to the flour and mix with chopsticks or fork. When you can handle it comfortably, knead the dough. Add oil and knead it again. Make a ball of dough, cover it with a wet cloth and let it sit for 30 minutes.

Remove cloth, knead once more. Roll into log 9″ long with diameter of 1½″ and slice into ½″ lengths. Roll each piece into a round shape with a 3½″ diameter.

Squeeze excess water from vegetables by hand. Add ginger juice, soy sauce and vegetables to the seitan. Mix together and add bread cubes (or sauteed rolled oats).

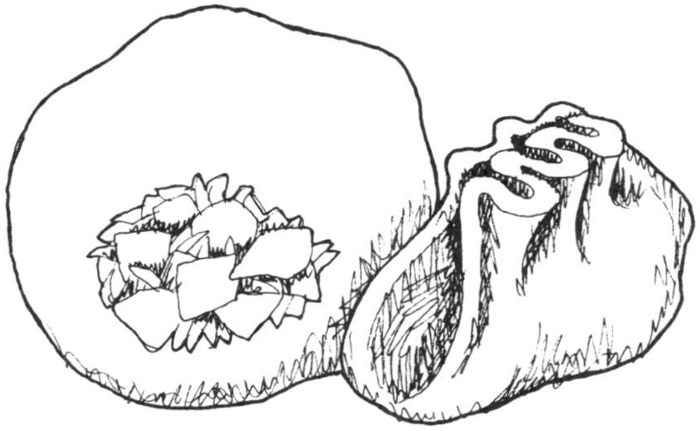

Fold each piece of dough gently — do not make a sharp crease when you fold. Leave the folded edge wide (about ¾″) and place 1 tsp. of the filling in each piece of dough. Flute dough on top, sealing it into gyoza shape.

Heat 2 Tbsp. oil in a heavy iron pan that has a cover. Place one layer of gyoza tightly in the pan and cook them until slightly brown (about 7 min.). Remove the cover and keep it in your hand; add 1 ladleful of boiling water (about ⅓ cup) and replace the cover immediately. The water will sizzle in the pan. Cook the gyoza 7 minutes more until all the water is evaporated. The gyoza will become more transparent.

Serve it with the brown side up, with lemon sauce.

Clear Party Soup with Vegetables 129.

3 cups soup stock (see 16. or 80a.)
2 cups water
1 tsp. sea salt
1 tsp. tamari soy sauce
5 pieces carrot, cut in flower shape
5 pieces of parsley
1 small pkg. somen (thin white noodles)
3 cups boiling water (for cooking somen noodles)

Tie each piece of parsley into a circle, loosely. Dip the tied parsley into the salted boiling water until its color changes and set it aside to cool.

Place the carrots in the same boiling water and cook them until they are tender (about 5 minutes). Strain and let them cool.

Add the water to the soup stock.

Cook the somen and rinse with cold water. Allow to cool. Pick up about 5 somen noodles, wrap them around your finger and place them in a bowl. Place 1 piece of carrot and one parsley circle along with noodles in each bowl.

Boil the mixed soup stock and vegetable water for 20 minutes and add soy sauce to season. Pour this hot stock over the noodles and vegetables. Serve it hot.

Rice Pie 130.

Filling: 2 cups fried rice (see 119.)
½ cup roasted pastry flour
1 cup water
½ tsp. sea salt

Pie shell: 3 cups whole wheat pastry flour
3 tsp. oil

Mix the ingredients for the pie shell. (Refer to 31.)

Mix the cold roasted flour with the salt and water. The consistency will be like tempura batter. Mix the rice into this and put it into the pie shell. (Please see 31. for apple pie baking.)

Bake at 450° for 45 minutes.

This recipe can be varied by adding leftover plain rice, vegetable stew or vegetable nitsuke.

Wild Scallion and Egg Nitsuke 131.

1 handful of wild scallions, cut 1″ koguchigiri
1 tsp. sesame oil
1 Tbsp. tamari soy sauce
1 egg, beaten

Saute the wild scallion on a high flame until the color changes. Add the soy sauce and cook uncovered for 5 minutes. Add the beaten egg, bring this to a boil, then shut off.

Wild scallions grow in many back yards. If you remove only the leaves above the root, they will grow for the entire season.

Amasake Cake

132.

3 cups whole wheat pastry flour, sifted
2 cups blended amasake, at body temperature (see 8.)
1 tsp. cinnamon
½ tsp. sea salt
3 Tbsp. corn oil

Yeast mixture:
1 cup warm water
½ tsp. yeast
5 heaping Tbsp. whole wheat pastry flour

Sift the flour 3 times. Add the oil, salt and cinnamon and mix these thoroughly. Rub the flour between the palms of your hands until all the oil lumps are mixed in.

Dissolve the yeast in warm water and let sit for 5 minutes. Then add the 5 heaping Tbsp. of flour. Let this mixture sit in a warm place until it bubbles (top of the stove over the pilot light is a good place).

Blend the amasake into the yeast mixture, then add the sifted flour, mixing it lightly with a wooden spoon. Do not stir it. Let this sit in a warm place in a covered bowl for 1 hour or until it has doubled in size. Then mix it again and let it sit for 50 minutes more.

Place the mixture in an oiled cake pan and bake it at 350° for 40 minutes. Remove the cake from the oven and let it cool. Then slice it in half and spread apple butter between the cut layers. Cover with frosting.

Amasake Cake Frosting

White:
1 cup blended amasake
1½ cups cold water
½ tsp. sea salt
2 level tsp. kanten powder *or* 1 Tbsp. kuzu or arrowroot flour
½ tsp. grated lemon peel

Add the water to the kanten, bring to boil in an uncovered pot with ½ tsp. salt. Cook for 10 minutes, skimming off the top bubbles, then stir in the amasake. Cook for 10 minutes more, still uncovered. Add the lemon peel, then set it aside to cool until the kanten partially thickens (about 20 minutes).

Dark:
1½ cups blended amasake
1 heaping Tbsp. yannoh (grain coffee)
2 tsp. kuzu or arrowroot flour, mixed with 2 Tbsp. water

For this frosting, heat the amasake and add the yannoh. Bring it to a boil, add the dissolved kuzu and boil it again. Cook 5 minutes, then set aside to cool.

Yam, Carrot Nitsuke 133.

3 6″ long yams, cut ½″ ichogiri
2 med. carrots, cut sainome (diced)
1 Tbsp. sesame oil
1 tsp. sea salt
¾ cup water

Heat the oil and saute the yams until slightly brown. Add the carrots and saute them a few minutes. Sprinkle on the salt and add the water. Bring them to a boil covered on a high flame, then cook them on a medium flame for 30 minutes or until the vegetables are tender, but still keep their shape.

Gomoku Rice 134.

3 cups cooked brown rice (see 1b.)
2 med. shiitake mushrooms, soaked and cut sengiri
3 12″ pieces of kampyo (dried gourd strips)
2 med. carrots, cut sasagaki
3 stalks parsley, blanched in boiling water, then minced
1 sheet nori, roasted and crushed
2 tsp. sesame oil
½ tsp. sea salt
1 Tbsp. tamari soy sauce

Soak the gourd strips by covering them with water. Cut them into ½″ pieces.

Heat the oil, saute the carrots a few minutes in a covered pan and add ¼ cup of boiling water. Sprinkle in ¼ tsp. salt and cook until they are tender but still keep their form.

In another pot, boil the sliced kampyo in its soaking water and cook it covered for 20 minutes or until it becomes transparent. Add ¼ tsp. salt and cook for another 20 minutes or until it is tender. If the kampyo is watery, remove the cover while it is cooking and let the water evaporate. Add 1 tsp. soy sauce and mix.

In another pot, bring the shiitake mushrooms to a boil in their soaking water. Add 1 tsp. soy sauce, cover the pot and cook the mushrooms for 15 minutes.

Place the cooked rice in a large bowl and mix in all the vegetables. Sprinkle the parsley and nori on top as condiments.

Variation: burdock, cut sasagaki
carrot, cut sasagaki
age, cut sengiri (see 64.)
green nori
fresh mushrooms, cut sengiri

The above vegetables can be substituted for those in the original recipe.

Amasake Yeasted Doughnuts 135.

2 cups blended amasake (see 8.)
6 cups whole wheat pastry flour
½ cup chestnut flour
1 tsp. cinnamon
3 Tbsp. corn oil

Yeast mixture:

½ to 1 tsp. yeast
½ cup warm water
2 heaping Tbsp. whole wheat pastry flour

Dissolve the yeast in the warm water and let it sit for 5 - 10 minutes in a warm place. Mix in the 2 Tbsp. of flour and let this sit another 5 - 10 minutes. Warm the amasake to room temperature, then stir in the yeast mixture.

In another bowl mix the 6 cups of flour with the oil. By hand, gently blend thoroughly. Mix together the contents of both bowls, add ½ cup warm water and knead like bread dough to blend it completely. Cover the bowl with a wet towel and set in a warm place until the dough doubles in size (about 4 hours). Punch down the dough and let it rise again for 1 hour.

Punch it down once more to remove the yeast gases. Roll out the dough on a floured board to a ½″ thickness. Make the doughnuts with a doughnut cutter. Place them on a wet cloth.

Heat fresh oil (2 - 3″ deep) in a deep frying pan over a high flame. Remove pan from flame and cool for 10 minutes, then heat it again over a medium flame. (Preheating the oil eliminates an excessive oil smell from the food.)

Drop the doughnuts into the oil without crowding them. They will drop to the bottom but in a few minutes will expand and rise. Increase the center hole in each doughnut by twirling a chopstick inside the hole, moving it around in the oil. When the color becomes golden, turn the doughnuts and fry the other side in the same manner.

Drain them in a strainer placed over a pan to catch the excess oil. Dust the hot doughnuts with a mixture of ½ cup chestnut flour and 1 tsp. cinnamon. Set aside on a cookie sheet covered with paper towels to cool.

Oatmeal 136.

2 cups rolled oats
6 cups cold water
½ tsp. sea salt

Roast the rolled oats in a dry iron or heavy stainless steel pot until they are fragrant. Use a flame slightly higher than medium.

Add 3 cups of cold water, allow the mixture to boil and add salt. Then add 3 more cups of water and bring to a boil again. Cook the oatmeal on a low flame for 1 hour without stirring. Stirring makes oatmeal stick to the pot.

Nuka Pickles

5 lbs. nuka (rice bran), about 25 cups
1½ cups sea salt
5 cups water
½ cup barley miso
Choice of vegetables

Suggested vegetables: daikon, daikon leaves, turnips, turnip leaves, carrots, celery, cabbage, Chinese cabbage, mustard greens, cucumber, watermelon rind, small winter squash, summer squash and eggplant.

Roast each cup of the nuka in an unoiled pan over a medium flame until it changes color slightly. Set it aside to cool. Bring the water to a boil, add the salt and let it cool. Place the nuka in a porcelain or wooden container, pour this cooled water over it and add the miso. The mixture should be soft, like miso paste.

At the start, the nuka paste is salty since the salt and nuka have not blended their flavors together. It is a somewhat unbalanced taste. For a couple of days, stir the nuka paste 3 times a day. This stirring will help to balance the taste. Also at this time, place 5 - 6 unused leaves such as outer cabbage leaves into the nuka paste; discard them every day for 3 days. After 10 days the nuka paste will have a balanced taste. At this point you are ready to make pickles.

If daikon or turnips are used, cut them in quarters or halves about 6″ long. If they are small, whole daikon can be used. Small cabbage can be pickled whole also. Use celery by the stalk, 1 or 2 at a time. Small whole carrots can be used. Chinese cabbage or any green leaves should be dried outdoors for 3 - 4 hours before being used. If you are pickling cabbage, eat the outer leaves first as they become soft; return the remainder of the head to the nuka paste for further pickling.

Vegetables are ready to serve when the color has changed or when they have become soft. Cucumbers require 24 hours, watermelon rind needs 5 - 6 hours, celery is ready overnight.

Remove vegetables from the pickling container and wash the excess nuka from them. Slice and serve, or keep them whole in a container in the refrigerator. Vegetables get saltier the longer they stay in the nuka paste.

As the nuka gets wetter, roast 2 cups of nuka and 1 Tbsp. of salt and mix these with the old nuka paste to return it to the original consistency. Egg shells placed in the nuka paste will keep pickles from souring. Leftover cooked rice, orange or tangerine skins and cooked fish bones can be put into the nuka paste for flavor. Remove after a few days. This also increases the mineral value of the pickles. During the summer, 5 - 6 chili peppers can be added to the paste to slow down fermentation and protect against insects laying eggs in the nuka. We recommend placing a cotton cloth under the cover of the pickling barrel to protect the nuka from flies and insects.

In Japan, nuka pickles are not eaten during the winter, but Americans can eat them all year ’round since they have such a yang constitution. For winter eating, add a wooden lid and a small stone for pressure to yangize the vegetables that are pickling.

Nuka paste can be saved for the next spring, if you choose not to make pickles in the winter or if you are going to be travelling. This is done by placing a strainer inside the nuka paste and removing all the liquid. Add 1 cup of salt and mix it well into the nuka. Press the nuka down and cover it with 1½ cups of salt. Over this place a wooden lid and seal it completely. Store this in a cool place. When spring comes or you want to make pickles again, repeat the same process as described earlier.

Note: If you are using pressure in the form of a wooden cover and stone, it will not be necessary to stir the nuka paste so often. Otherwise, be sure to stir it occasionally since nuka needs oxygen.

Vegetable Kabobs with Lemon Miso Sauce 138.

1 small cauliflower
10 string beans or 1 bunch broccoli
2 carrots
3 stalks celery
8 cups boiling water
1 Tbsp. sea salt

Cook the vegetables whole, separately, in boiling salted water in an uncovered pot on a high flame. Cook the cauliflower about 7 minutes, the other vegetables until they are tender. Remove from the water and let them cool.

Separate the cauliflower and broccoli into flowerettes. Cut the string beans in half and cut the celery and carrots into 1½″ pieces (wagiri).

On a bamboo skewer place pieces of carrot, celery, string bean and cauliflower. Place the cauliflower so that it covers the skewer point. It will look like a flower on the end of the skewer.

Sauce: 1 heaping Tbsp. rice miso
1 heaping Tbsp. barley miso
⅔ cup water from the cooked vegetables
1 tsp. lemon rind, grated
1 Tbsp. lemon juice

Bring the water to a boil, add the miso and shut off the heat. Add the lemon rind, let the sauce cool completely and then add the lemon juice. Serve this sauce with the vegetable kabobs.

Dandelion and Cabbage Nitsuke 139.

1 cabbage, cut thin sengiri
7 dandelion plants - roots, minced; leaves cut ¼″ koguchigiri
1 Tbsp. sesame oil
1 Tbsp. tamari soy sauce

Heat the oil and saute the dandelion roots on a medium flame for 10 minutes in a covered pan. Add the leaves and saute them until their color changes. Add the cabbage and when its color changes, add the soy sauce and cook the nitsuke until tender in a covered pan. This will take about 10 minutes.

Wild vegetables cannot be eaten in excess, so our proportions are 3 parts cultivated vegetables to 1 part wild plants.

Dried Daikon Nitsuke 140.

1 cup dried daikon (available at Oriental food stores) and soaking water
1 tsp. sesame oil
¼ tsp. sea salt
2 tsp. tamari soy sauce

Soak the daikon for 20 minutes in the water. Strain and squeeze out the water through a cotton cloth and reserve it. Cut the daikon into 1″ strips.

Heat the oil, add the daikon and saute it for 5 minutes. Add the soaking water and bring to a boil on a high flame. Continue cooking the daikon for 45 minutes on a low flame, or until it is tender. Add more water if necessary.

Add the salt and cook the nitsuke 20 minutes longer. Add the soy sauce and serve.

Condiment Pickles 141.

½ cup Chinese cabbage, leafy green part
¼ cup old cucumber pickles
1 tsp. ginger pickles or minced ginger
2 heaping Tbsp. scallions, cut thin koguchigiri
1 heaping Tbsp. bonita flakes
2 tsp. tamari soy sauce

Chop the Chinese cabbage and the cucumber pickles finely. Wash them well in a strainer and squeeze out all the excess water. Add the ginger pickles, scallions, bonita flakes and soy sauce and mix together.

These pickles sharpen the appetite.

Variation: 1 cup scallions, cut thin koguchigiri
2 heaping Tbsp. bonita flakes
1 - 2 Tbsp. tamari soy sauce or 1 Tbsp. barley miso

Mix all ingredients together.

This is a good condiment to improve the appetite.

Baked Apples 142.

10 small apples
½ cup water

Remove the core of the apples and place them in a glass baking dish so that all the apples are tightly packed together.

Add the water and bake them for 2 hours at 450° or until the apples are tender. When serving them, pour some of the syrup that has collected in the dish over the apples.

Pour hot bancha tea into the baking dish to wash out the extra apple syrup. This makes a nice sweet drink.

Umeboshi Dressing 143.

5 umeboshi (salt plums)
2 Tbsp. oil
1 onion, minced
1 tsp. lemon rind, grated

Remove the pits from the salt plums. Use either a blender or a suribachi to blend the oil with the salt plums. Add the minced onion, let the dressing sit for 20 minutes and then mix it with the salad.

If necessary, add more salt.

When you mix the dressing with the salad, add in the lemon rind.

Squash and Dried Fruit Kanten 144.

1½ cups dried prunes, pitted
1½ cups raisins
4 cups water, for soaking the above
2 cups baked squash, cut into bite-size pieces
2 heaping Tbsp. kanten powder
or about 4 kanten bars
7 cups cold water

Soak the fruit for 2 hours in the water. Bring it to a boil and cook for 20 minutes. Blend in a blender.

Mix the kanten powder with water. Bring it to a boil and cook 15 minutes. Skim the white bubbles off the top and throw them away. Mix in the blended fruits and squash and boil the kanten 5 minutes.

Place it in a mold or dish to cool and become firm.

Note: When cooking the kanten, never cover.

Sweet Brown Rice and Azuki Bean 145.

8 cups sweet brown rice
2 cups azuki beans
10 cups water

After washing the beans and rice, soak them together in the water for 24 hours.

Cook them together in a pressure cooker for about 40 minutes on a flame slightly higher than medium. When pressure top begins to jiggle, turn the flame to low and cook 20 minutes more.

Shut off the heat and let pot sit for 1 hour before serving.

Mix top and bottom, then serve hot or warm with gomashio.

Norimake Sushi 146.

5 sheets nori
8 cups hot cooked rice
3 carrots
1 bunch spinach
2 Tbsp. umeboshi juice, or lemon juice
1 tsp. tamari soy sauce
½ tsp. salt

Omelette:
4 eggs
3 Tbsp. soup stock or sake or water
½ tsp. sea salt
½ tsp. tamari soy sauce

Make umeboshi juice by boiling 7 salt plums in ½ cup water; cook for 20 minutes. Mix this umeboshi juice or lemon juice with hot rice, then let the rice cool.

Note: In the summertime, if you have shiso leaves, mince these and mix them with hot rice instead of umeboshi or lemon juice.

Cut the carrots into lengthwise strips about ⅜″ thick. Saute them lightly in oil for 10 minutes, then add soy sauce and salt. Cover and cook this on low heat for 10 minutes more. Uncover, stir the carrots gently and cook until tender.

Boil the spinach in salted water, uncovered, until it is soft but still bright green in color. Then remove from the water and spread it out on a strainer to cool. Squeeze water from the spinach and sprinkle with soy sauce.

Mix omelette ingredients. Heat a small amount of oil in a medium-sized frying pan (square-shaped is better). Then pour in ⅔ of this mixture and cook uncovered until the top is set. Fold it carefully into thirds. Leaving this in the pan, oil the rest of the pan and pour the remaining egg mixture in. Cook until it is set and fold it over twice. There should then be 6 layers. Cool, then cut the omelettes into strips ⅜″ wide.

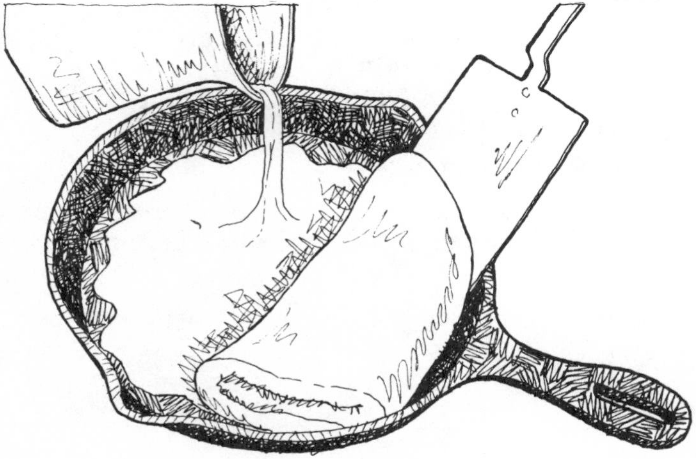

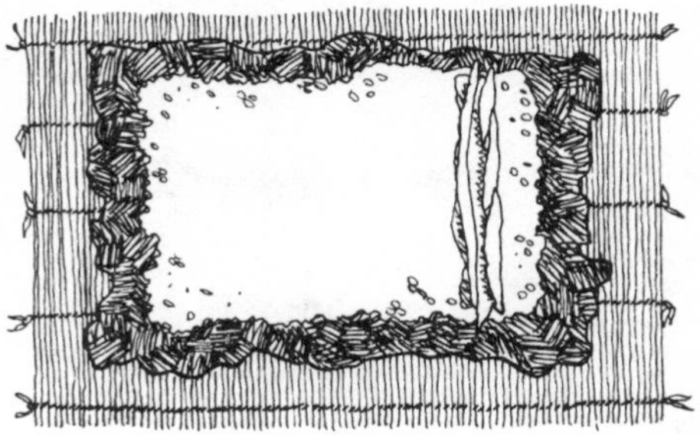

On a clean bamboo sushi mat lay 1 sheet of nori. Wet your hands with a small amount of lemon or umeboshi juice and spread the rice over the nori to within 1″ of the edge — a little more than 1″ at the top and a little less at the bottom. Two inches from the bottom edge, make a groove in the rice and in this place 2 carrot pieces, 1 strip of omelette and 3 spinach strips. Roll up the rice with the bamboo mat like a cigarette, pressing firmly all

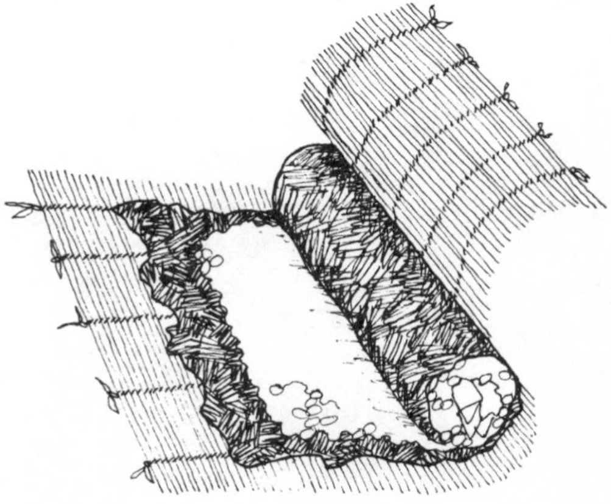

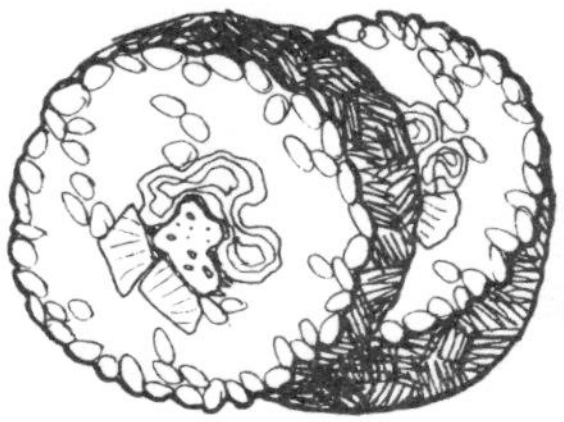

the time to keep a uniform shape and size. Use a sharp, wet knife to cut the roll into slices about ¾″ thick. Arrange them on a plate with the flat side down.

These are very good to take on picnics.

Piroshki 147.

7 cups whole wheat pastry flour
½ tsp. yeast
2½ cups warm water
1 Tbsp. sea salt
1 Tbsp. oil

Filling 1: 1 cup cooked hijiki (see 186.)

2: 2 cups sliced cabbage
½ tsp. sea salt
1 heaping Tbsp. mayonnaise (see 76.)
2 tsp. arrowroot flour

Mix the cabbage and salt and knead together in a suribachi until the cabbage is soft. Squeeze out all the water from the cabbage, mix it with mayonnaise and sprinkle in the arrowroot.

Dissolve the yeast in warm water. After 5 minutes add the oil and salt, then mix in the flour and knead the dough until it has an ear lobe consistency. Let this sit overnight or for at least 4 hours in a warm place until it has doubled in size.

Roll the dough into a broomstick-like shape with a 1½″ diameter and cut into 1″ thick sections. Roll out each section to a 4″ diameter and place 1 heaping tsp. of the hijiki or cabbage filling in the center. Fold the dough in half, seal it and, if you wish, make a pattern on the edge of the dough.

Deep-fry the piroshki on a medium high flame until golden brown. Drain and serve.

Note: Be sure that each one is sealed tightly, otherwise it will open up in the hot oil.

Variation: Use sauteed cabbage mixed with cooked okara as a stuffing.

Hijiki Nori Nitsuke 148.

½ cup cooked hijiki (see 186.)
1 pkg. of nori, 10 sheets
2 - 3 Tbsp. tamari soy sauce

Tear the nori into 1″ squares and soak it in 2 cups of water for 20 minutes.

Bring this to a boil and cook for 20 minutes. Add the soy sauce and cooked hijiki and cook it for another 20 minutes.

If there is too much water, boil off the excess.

This dish is appealing even to those who don't care for hijiki.

Ohagi

149.

5 cups sweet brown rice
5 cups water

Topping 1: 1 cup green peas, dried and whole
1 cup dried chestnuts or ½ cup yinnie syrup
1 tsp. sea salt

2: ½ cup brown sesame seeds
1 Tbsp. tamari soy sauce

3: 6 sheets nori

Wash the sweet rice and soak it overnight with 5 cups of water. Pressure cook this using a flame slightly higher than medium until the weight jiggles (about 30 minutes), then lower the flame and cook it another 20 minutes. Turn off the flame and let the rice sit 45 minutes.

Pound the rice with a wooden mallet for about 10 minutes. Wet your hands, shape the rice into rectangles and cover with toppings.

Green Pea and Chestnut Topping

Wash the chestnuts and green peas. If possible, remove the skins from the chestnuts. Soak 4 - 5 hours in 4 cups of water, then pressure cook 45 minutes. When the pressure comes down, add 1 tsp. salt and cook 30 minutes. Mash them slightly with a potato masher or something similar. Leave the cover off and let this cool.

If using yinnie syrup instead of chestnuts, pressure cook green peas; when pressure comes down, add ½ cup yinnie syrup and cook for 10 minutes. Add 1 tsp. salt, cook for 10 more minutes, then mash and cool.

Sesame Seed Topping

Wash the sesame seeds. Strain and roast them in a dry pan on a medium flame until they smoke slightly - about 15 minutes. Place them in a suribachi, sprinkle on 1 Tbsp. soy sauce and grind them gently until the soy sauce and sesame seeds are thoroughly mixed.

Nori Topping

Take 2 sheets of nori, place the shiny sides together and roast them over a medium flame until they turn green. Place nori in a cotton towel and crush it into small pieces. Place this crushed nori on a flat plate.

Use these different toppings to cover the rice rectangles. You will have 3 colors — green, brown and black.

March 21 and September 23 mark the equinoxes - special days of the year when the Japanese traditionally honor and pray to their ancestors. Ohagi is a special food offering to the ancestors.

Parsnip Yam Nitsuke

150.

2 med. parsnips, diced ¼″
4 med. yams, cut 1″ koguchigiri (cut in half if too large)
1 Tbsp. oil
1 tsp. sea salt
¼ cup boiling water

Heat the oil and saute the yams on a medium flame for 10 minutes. When they are slightly brown, add the parsnips and saute them a few minutes. Sprinkle with salt and add the boiling water. Bring this to a boil, lower the flame and cook 20 - 30 minutes, until yams are tender.

Stuffed Cabbage with White Sauce 151.

10 cabbage leaves
2″ × 2″ piece of dashi kombu, cut with 1½″ slits, not completely through (comb-like)
1¼ tsp. sea salt
⅓ cup white bechamel sauce (using unbleached white flour)
1 Tbsp. tamari soy sauce
1 heaping Tbsp. fresh minced parsley
10 carrot croquettes

Croquettes:
½ cup grated carrot
¼ cup minced onion
½ cup whole wheat flour
1 Tbsp. buckwheat flour
½ tsp. sea salt
oil for deep-frying

Mix ingredients for carrot croquettes. The carrot, onion, salt and flours will all stick together. Shape into 10 small rectangles and deep-fry them until they are crisp.

Cook the cabbage leaves in boiling water with 1 tsp. salt until they are slightly tender. Let them cool, then remove the hard part at the bottom of the leaf which was connected to the core (the area shaped like a triangle).

Place a carrot croquette in each leaf. Wrap up the leaf and secure with a toothpick. Place the kombu at the bottom of a pan and place the cabbage rolls on top. Cover them with the water left from cooking the cabbage and bring to a boil on a high flame. Add ¼ tsp. salt and 1 Tbsp. soy sauce and cook for 20 minutes. Make white bechamel sauce (using recipe 37a.) and pour this white sauce over the cabbage rolls. Bring to a boil for a few minutes, sprinkle with parsley and serve hot.

Apple Butter 152.

10 apples

Grate 2 apples and then cut the remaining 8 into very thin slices.

In a heavy stainless steel pot, place the grated apples on the bottom and the sliced apples on top. Push them down tightly. Cook on a low flame for 50 minutes in a covered pot.

When the juice comes out of the apples, turn the flame up to medium low. As the juice comes out, mix the apples from the top to the bottom and cook them until they are very tender.

If there is too much juice, take off the cover and cook away the excess water.

Cooking apples on a low flame for a long time makes them more yang and brings out their sweet flavor.

Rye Bread 153.

4 cups whole wheat flour
3 cups rye flour
1 cup brown rice flour
½ tsp. yeast
1 cup warm water
1 Tbsp. oil
1 Tbsp. sea salt
1 tsp. caraway seeds
2 cups warm water

Dissolve the yeast in 1 cup of warm water and let it sit for 5 minutes. Add the oil and salt and mix in all dry ingredients. Add 2 cups of warm water, knead the dough to an ear lobe consistency and let sit overnight in a warm place. The dough will rise a little.

Oil and heat the bread pans on top of the stove. Place the dough in the pans and cut down the center about 1″ deep. Place these in a cold (not preheated) oven and bake at 450° for 1 hour.

Vegetables with Macaroni 154.

10 flowerettes of cauliflower
3 stalks broccoli, cut into flowerettes
2 onions, cut ¼″ mawashigiri
1 carrot, cut ichogiri
3″ of daikon, cut ichogiri
2 cups macaroni
½ cup bechamel sauce (see 37a.)
1 Tbsp. sesame oil
1 Tbsp. tamari soy sauce

Cook the macaroni in 8 cups of boiling water. Strain and reserve the water. Boil the cauliflower in this water for 5 minutes, then set it aside to cool. Cook the broccoli with the same water, uncovered.

Heat the oil and saute the onions until they are transparent. Add the daikon and the carrot. Saute these for 3 minutes, cover with water and cook for 20 minutes.

Add the vegetable water and the bechamel sauce. Add the macaroni and bring it to a boil. Add the soy sauce and bring to a boil again. Add the cooked cauliflower and broccoli and serve the dish hot.

Vegetable Fritters 155.

1 cup carrot, cut thin hasugiri
1 cup burdock, cut thin hasugiri
½ cup whole wheat flour
3 Tbsp. oil
1 tsp. sea salt
1 Tbsp. tamari soy sauce

Place the flour in a plastic bag. Add the burdock and shake the bag vigorously. Remove the burdock from the bag. Heat the oil in a skillet. Place the floured burdock in the pan, cover it and cook over a medium heat for 5 minutes.

Place the carrots in the same bag and shake them. Add these to the burdock when it has become soft. Cook until carrots are soft. Then add the salt and soy sauce. Sprinkle ¼ cup water onto the vegetables in a spiral motion, beginning at the outer edge of the skillet. Add ¼ cup more water if necessary and cook the vegetables until they are tender.

Adjust the seasoning and remove the fritters from the pan.

Horsetail Nitsuke 156.

1 handful horsetail
1 Tbsp. sesame oil
1 Tbsp. tamari soy sauce

Clean the horsetail, removing the top and flower parts and the outer skin on the brown areas. Cut it into 2″ koguchigiri pieces.

Heat the oil and saute the horsetail on a medium flame about 7 minutes. Add the soy sauce and cook it until it is tender — about 7 minutes more.

Horsetail has the highest calcium content of all the vegetables. For any calcium deficiency, weak bones or weak lungs this is an excellent dish.

Eggplant Mustard Pickles 157.

2 lbs. small young eggplant
4 Tbsp. sea salt
½ cup boiling water
1 cup rice koji
1 cup mustard powder
⅔ cup tamari soy sauce
5 Tbsp. yinnie syrup
1 Tbsp. sea salt
½ cup soup stock (see 16. or 80a.)

Wash the eggplants and cut (halve) them lengthwise. Salt them with the 4 Tbsp. salt and put them in a vegetable press with ½ cup of water around the edges. Press them down hard for 2 - 3 days. Remove the eggplant and cut into strips ½″ wide. Squeeze the strips firmly to remove the excess water.

Mix soy sauce, yinnie syrup and salt and bring this to a boil. When it has cooled, pour it into a bowl and saturate the eggplant with this sauce.

Add the boiling water to the mustard powder until it is thick and creamy. Put thin layers of this mustard mixture on the bottom and sides of a small bowl. Cover this with rice paper. Fill the bowl with boiling water and place 2 - 3 burning red wooden coals in it. After 10 minutes throw out the coals and the water. Slowly remove the rice paper from inside the bowl, and turn the bowl upside down for about 20 minutes. Then thoroughly mix the mustard in the bowl, add the rice koji to the mustard and mix well. Add the cold soup stock and mix thoroughly.

Spread a thin layer of this mixture on the bottom of a clean, dry earthenware container. Snugly place the eggplant strips in layers 1½″ thick into it. Continue making layers of eggplant with mustard sauce between them. Finish with mustard sauce on top.

Cover this with rice paper, then a clay cover and seal it with tape. Keep it in a cool place. You can eat these pickles in a week to a month.

These pickles are good for diarrhea.

Sake-Kasu Pickles

158.

5 lbs. pickling cucumbers (or 2 lbs. shiro-uri, Japanese cucumbers)
2 lbs. turnips
2 eggplants
1 daikon
2 - 3 cups sea salt
4 - 5 lbs. sake-kasu (leftover from making sake, available at Japanese stores)

Wash the vegetables. Mix them with 10% of their weight in salt and put them in a container. Press them with a very heavy stone so that liquid comes to the top after 24 hours.

Remove them from the container and keep them dry for half a day indoors.

On the bottom of a clean large crock, spread a 1″ thick layer of the kasu and put a layer of the pressed vegetables on top of it. Repeat this layering until the crock or keg is full, ending with a layer of kasu. Cover with cotton cloth and crock cover, then seal. After 1 month the pickles will be ready to eat.

This process can be repeated using the same kasu.

Koi-Koku *(Carp Soup)*

159.

1 carp, 1 - 2 lbs.
5 - 7 cups burdock, cut sasagaki (the cut burdock should be 3 times the volume of the carp)
2 tsp. sesame oil
⅓ to ½ cup barley miso

Clean the carp and carefully remove the gall bladder; it is bitter, so don't break it. If you should, wash the area immediately with bancha tea. Do not remove the scales. Cut the fish in ½″ slices.

Heat the oil and saute the burdock until its smell is gone. Add the carp and cover with water. Put some used bancha tea leaves in a bag tied at the top and immerse it in the water. Bring the soup to a boil and then simmer 4 - 5 hours, until the bones of the fish are soft.

Remove the bag of tea leaves.

Mix the miso with a little water, add this to the soup and simmer one hour more. (If you pressure-cook the carp, cook for 2 hours or more depending on the size of the fish. After the pressure has gone down, take out the tea bag and add the miso.)

When you serve this soup add a pinch of grated ginger on top.

Use the whole fish, including the head. Remove only the gall bladder.

If the fish is fresh, it should be kept alive in clean water for a day to clean out its intestines. If you are not able to do this, the intestines should be discarded. Carp live at the bottom of the lake and their intestines are full of mud.

Whole Wheat Noodle Salad with Sesame Dressing 160.

2 oz. whole wheat spaghetti noodles
1 med. carrot, cut thin sengiri
1½ heads of lettuce, torn into 1″ squares
2 stalks of celery, cut thin hasugiri
¼ cantaloupe, cut ¼″ thick and in ½″ squares (optional)
2 tsp. sesame oil
1¼ tsp. sea salt

Dressing:
3 salt plums (remove pits and grind in a suribachi)
1 Tbsp. sesame butter
5 Tbsp. boiling water that has been slightly cooled
1 Tbsp. tamari soy sauce
1 med. onion, cut mijingiri

Heat the oil and saute the carrots on a medium flame in a covered pot until they are tender. Add ¼ tsp. of salt and set aside to cool.

Bring to a boil 4 cups of water with 1 tsp. salt. Break the noodles into 5 pieces and add them to the boiling water. Bring to a boil, add cold water and boil again. Turn off the heat and let it sit a few minutes.

Strain and reserve the water for making bread.

Wash the noodles in cold water repeatedly until they are cold, and strain off all the water.

Mix together the salt plums, sesame butter, soy sauce and water. Add the onions and let this sit for 30 minutes. If necessary add more water. The dressing should be soft but not runny.

Mix the noodles, vegetables and fruit together. Mix in the dressing and serve the salad immediately.

Amasake Cake with Fruit and Nuts 161.

6 cups whole wheat pastry flour
2 cups uncooked oatmeal
2 cups sliced walnuts
1 cup currants
6 Tbsp. oil
2 cups blended amasake (see 8.)
2 cups warm water
2 tsp. sea salt
1 tsp. yeast

Dissolve the yeast in warm water. Let it sit for 5 minutes, then mix in the warmed amasake.

Sift the flour 3 times and mix it with the oatmeal. Add the salt and oil to this mixture. Be sure to distribute the oil evenly throughout the dry ingredients. Add the walnuts and currants and mix in the yeast batter. Now mix all the ingredients together with a wooden spoon; this will form a loose batter. Cover and place it in a warm spot to rise for 2 - 3 hours or until it is double in size.

Punch down the dough and stir it thoroughly. Cover and let it rise again, about 1 hour.

Oil a cake pan, pour the batter into it and place it into a cold oven. Turn the oven on to 450° and bake for 40 minutes.

Seitan Goma Rice 162.

8 cups brown rice
2 cups seitan (see 87a.)
½ cup white sesame seeds (see 109.)
9 cups water

Wash the sesame seeds (as in 109.).

Wash the rice (see 1b.).

Mix all the ingredients and cook as in 1b.

Sauteed Onion, Potato and Green Pepper 163.

2 med. onions, diced
3 med. potatoes, cut sengiri
3 green peppers, diced
2 Tbsp. oil
1 tsp. sea salt
2 tsp. tamari soy sauce

In a heavy frying pan, saute the potatoes. Keep a lid on the pan while they are cooking. Saute them on each side for 5 minutes. Add the onions and green pepper and continue to saute until the green pepper becomes bright green.

Add the salt and soy sauce and cook the vegetables 5 minutes more. Serve them hot.

Noodle Croquettes 164.

2 cups leftover fried noodles (29.)
1 cup rice kayu or leftover rice cream (96. or 49.)
½ cup whole wheat pastry flour
1 heaping Tbsp. minced seitan
½ cup bread crumbs, corn meal or sweet rice flour
2 Tbsp. corn oil

Mix all the above ingredients together except the last two.

Shape into croquettes and cover them with bread crumbs, corn meal or sweet rice flour and let them sit for 5 minutes.

Heat up a frying pan and add the 2 Tbsp. of oil. Fry the croquettes in a covered pan on a medium flame until both sides are slightly brown — about 7 minutes on each side.

Serve them hot.

Note: If you use sweet brown rice flour to dust the croquettes, it will give them a nice white color.

Raisin Cake

165.

4 cups yellow raisins
6 cups water
4 cups unbleached white flour
2 Tbsp. oil
½ tsp. sea salt
½ tsp. yeast
½ cup warm water
2 heaping Tbsp. unbleached white flour
1 heaping Tbsp. arrowroot flour

Soak the raisins overnight in 6 cups of water, then pressure-cook them for 20 minutes. Place them in a blender and blend slowly so that the raisins still have some shape.

Dissolve the yeast in warm water and let it sit for 5 minutes. Add the 2 Tbsp. of flour and let sit about 5 minutes more until the mixture bubbles. Then add 2 cups of the warm raisin puree.

Mix the oil, salt and 4 cups of flour in another bowl, add the yeast mixture to this and stir it with a wooden spoon. Cover and let it sit for 2 - 3 hours in a warm place. When it doubles in size, punch it down and stir. Cover and let it rise again for 1 hour.

Place the dough in 2 oiled cake pans and place these in a cold oven. Turn the temperature to 400° and bake them for 30 minutes.

Frosting

To the remaining raisin puree add 1 heaping Tbsp. of arrowroot which has been dissolved in cold water. Cook this until it thickens. Let it cool and use it for the cake frosting.

Roast Turkey with Stuffing

166.

25 lb. turkey
4 tsp. sea salt
1 lemon

Marinade:
⅔ cup tamari soy sauce
1 cup water or ½ cup sake
3 tsp. sea salt
4 Tbsp. ginger juice (grated and squeezed fresh ginger)

Remove the fat pieces of the turkey near its tail and save them for gravy. Wipe the turkey inside and out with a paper towel. Take out all the internal blood clots. Slice the lemon in half and rub it all over the outside of the turkey. Then rub on the salt, inside and out. Let it sit for 30 minutes. This removes the bloody taste of the bird.

Wipe off all the excess salt with a paper towel. Mix the marinade sauce and marinate the turkey, brushing the marinade over the turkey 3 to 4 times during a 2 - 3 hour period.

Stuffing:
5 cups roasted brown rice
10 cups boiling water
1½ cups minced onions
1½ cups minced celery
1 cup shiitake mushrooms, soaked in warm water for 30 min., then sliced thin
2 Tbsp. sesame oil
3 tsp. sea salt
10 cups bread, diced in ½″ squares (let bread sit in oven 1 hour to dry, on low heat)

Mix the rice and boiling water and cook this in a preheated oven at 350° for 1 hour.

Heat the oil and saute the onion, mushrooms and celery. Add the salt and continue to saute them for 20 minutes on a medium high flame. Mix these vegetables with the cooked rice and allow to cool. Then mix in the dried bread cubes.

Place the stuffing in the turkey and close up the opening with skewers and cotton thread. After stuffing the turkey, turn the oven to 450° and bake it for about 45 minutes until it is golden brown. Remove the turkey from the oven, let it cool slightly, then wrap it twice in silver foil. Roast it with the chest up on a roasting rack for 7 hours at 250°.

Turn off the heat and let the turkey sit in the oven for 1 hour. When it has cooled, carefully remove the foil; there will be a lot of juice and oil in the foil. Save this for the gravy.

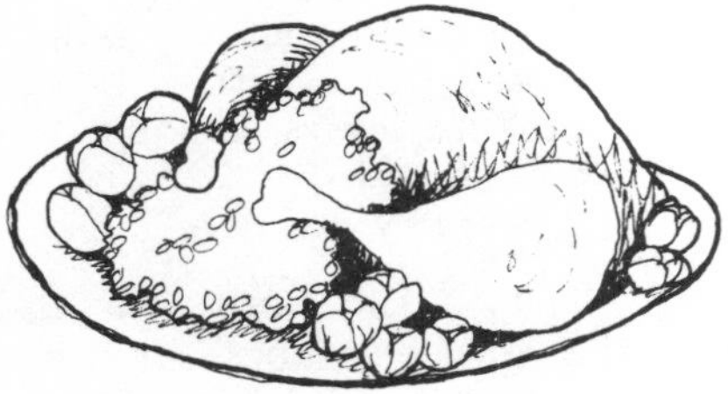

Turkey Gravy 166a.

Place the fat pieces which you removed from the turkey in a heavy frying pan. Heat them and let the fat melt. Cook this about 20 minutes on a medium flame.

Add 4 cups of whole wheat pastry flour and saute on a medium flame until the flour is brown. Set this aside to cool and mix it with 10 cups of water. Bring it to a boil, stirring frequently. Add 3 Tbsp. of salt, the juice from the cooked turkey and any extra marinade sauce. Boil this for 20 minutes and serve it hot.

Sesame Spaghetti with Oyster Sauce *(Serves 20)* 167.

3 lbs. sesame spaghetti
20 oysters
1 lb. fresh mushrooms, washed in salted water and sliced thin
4 med. onions, cut mijingiri
1 bunch parsley, cut mijingiri (separate stems and leaves)
3 Tbsp. sesame oil
4 tsp. sea salt
1/3 cup tamari soy sauce

Wash the oysters in a strainer. First sprinkle with 2 tsp. salt, then set strainer with oysters in a bowl of water and shake. This way you can wash gently and not break the oysters.

Boil 8 cups of water, add the oysters and cook them a few minutes uncovered. Strain them and save the excess water. When the oysters are cool, cut them into small pieces.

Heat up 2 Tbsp. oil and saute the oysters over a high flame for a few minutes. Remove them from the pan. Add the remaining Tbsp. oil and saute the onion, mushrooms and parsley stems. Add the 2 tsp. salt and the reserved water and cook the sauce for 20 minutes.

Add the chopped oysters, minced parsley leaves and the soy sauce. Bring this to a boil and serve over cooked spaghetti.

Baked Potatoes 168.

20 potatoes, medium size
½ lb. butter

Wash the potatoes and make 3 - 4 holes in each one with a fork. Bake them in a 450° oven for 2 hours or until they are soft throughout.

Serve them with butter and salt.

Fruit Punch 169.

3 med. apples, cut into ½″ cubes
4 oranges, peeled and cut into ½″ cubes
1 basket strawberries
1 lb. seedless green grapes
8 cups apple juice

Mix all ingredients and serve the punch chilled.

Rice Bread 170.

10 cups whole wheat flour
5 cups brown rice flour
5 cups warm water
4 tsp. sea salt
3 Tbsp. oil

Mix the flours, salt and oil thoroughly. Then add the water and knead the dough until it is an ear lobe consistency.

Divide it into 4 loaves of bread and place into bread pans. Make a cut down the center of each loaf about ½″ deep.

Bake the bread in a 300° oven for 1½ hours.

Millet Kayu 171.

2 cups millet
8 cups boiling water
½ tsp. sea salt

Wash the millet and place it in a pressure cooker. Add the boiling water and pressure-cook it with salt for 20 minutes.

Shut off the heat and allow the pressure to come down. Mix the millet from top to bottom and serve hot.

Whole Wheat Flour Tortilla *(Chapati)* 172.

6 cups whole wheat pastry flour
2½ tsp. sea salt
2½ cups boiling water
2 Tbsp. oil
1 large onion, cut very thin mawashigiri
1 carrot, cut sengiri
5 cabbage leaves, cut into pieces 1½″ long and shredded
½ tsp. curry powder

Mix 1½ tsp. salt with the flour and add the water. Knead it until the dough reaches ear lobe consistency. Roll it out into logs 1″ in diameter, then cut them into 1″ pieces and roll them out to a diameter of 4 - 5″.

Heat the oil in a frying pan and cook the chapatis on both sides until the color changes slightly to light golden. Another method of cooking is to heat a metal Japanese toaster on top of the stove using a medium flame. Place the chapati on top of the toaster and cook it on both sides until it puffs up a little, then remove it from the heat. Brush them lightly with sesame oil on one side only.

Saute the onion in 1 Tbsp. of oil, then add the cabbage and carrot. When the vegetables are tender, season them with 1 tsp. salt and the curry powder.

Break open the chapatis with your fingers and stuff with this filling.

Mrs. Lima Ohsawa said this sandwich is a staple food in India.

Horsetail Onion Roll 173.

Horsetail nitsuke (for preparation see 156.)
Onion nitsuke (use 35., substituting tamari for miso)
Chapati dough (see 172.)
oil for tempura

Make a dough using whole wheat pastry flour and a small amount of water and salt (same as 172., chapati dough).

Roll it out to a ⅛″ thickness and place it on a bamboo sushi mat. Spread a layer of horsetail and onion nitsuke over the dough, leaving a 1″ border on two sides. Roll the mat (like a jelly roll) and seal the ends of the dough with a little water.

Deep-fry the whole roll in tempura oil. Drain and cut it into ¾″ pieces and serve.

Raisin Roll 174.

½ cup raisins
2 cups sliced apples
1 cup sliced peaches
½ cup raisin water
1 cup water
½ tsp. cinnamon

Dough: ¼ cup oatmeal
2¾ cups unbleached white flour
¼ tsp. sea salt
3 Tbsp. corn oil
2½ cups boiling water

Cook the raisins in 1 cup of water for 20 minutes. Strain, then save the water.

Mix the fruit and cinnamon with ½ cup of raisin water and cook uncovered for 5 minutes. Then allow it to cool.

Mix all the dry ingredients for the dough. Add the boiling water, knead the dough and let it sit for 20 minutes, covered with a damp cloth.

Roll into an 8″ × 16″ rectangle on a floured board and cover it with the fruit filling. Leave 1″ around the edges. Roll up the dough and bake it at 350° for 30 minutes.

Broccoli and Collard Green Nitsuke 175.

- 1 bunch broccoli (separate flowers, cut stem ¼″ koguchigiri)
- 1 bunch collard greens, cut 1″ koguchigiri
- 2 Tbsp. oil
- ½ tsp. sea salt
- 2 Tbsp. tamari soy sauce

Heat the oil and saute the broccoli stems until they are bright green. Add the collard greens and saute them until they are bright green. Then add the broccoli flowers, cover and saute for 5 minutes.

Add the salt and soy sauce and stir the nitsuke lightly. Cover and cook it on a low flame for 10 minutes. When the juice comes out of the vegetables, cook them 15 - 20 minutes longer on a medium flame until they are tender.

Lentil Soup 176.

- 1 cup lentils
- 3 med. onions, cut thin mawashigiri
- 1 med. carrot, cut ⅛″ ichogiri
- ½ stalk celery, cut ¼″ sainome (diced)
- 1 Tbsp. sesame oil
- 4 cups boiling water
- 1 tsp. sea salt
- 1 tsp. tamari soy sauce

Soak the lentils in 2 cups of water for at least 2 hours. Cook them until they are tender, in a pressure cooker — 30 minutes. In a regular pot, cook for 1 hour.

In another pot, heat the oil and saute the onions on a medium flame until they are slightly brown. Add the carrots and saute them a few minutes, then add the celery and saute it until its color changes. Add the boiling water and let the vegetables come to a boil. Cook them for 20 minutes on a low flame.

Add the cooked lentils and the salt and continue cooking for 20 minutes more. Add soy sauce to taste.

Buckwheat Dumpling Miso Soup 177.

- 1 med. onion, cut thin mawashigiri
- 6″ piece of daikon, cut ⅛″ ichogiri
- daikon leaves, cut ¼″ koguchigiri
- 5 string beans, cut 1½″ koguchigiri
- 1 shiitake mushroom
- 1 Tbsp. sesame oil
- 1 heaping Tbsp. miso
- 8 cups boiling water

Dumplings:
- 1 cup buckwheat flour
- ⅓ cup cold water

Soak the mushroom in water until it is soft, about 20 minutes, then cut it ¼″ sengiri. Save its water for the soup.

Heat the oil and saute the onions until they are transparent. Add the mushroom, daikon leaves, string beans and daikon in that order. Saute each vegetable a few minutes before adding the next one. Add the boiling water and reserved mushroom soaking water and cook this until the vegetables are tender.

Mix the flour and water for dumplings. Drop them into the soup by heaping teaspoonfuls. When the dumplings float to the top of the soup, turn off the flame.

Dilute the miso with some of the soup stock and add it to the soup. Stir well and serve hot.

Note: Leftover brown rice or cooked cereal can be mixed into the dumpling batter. This will give it a light and delicious taste.

Sweet Potato Baked in Ashes 178.

10 sweet potatoes

Wash the sweet potatoes and wrap each one with 2 layers of wet newspapers.

After any kind of fire which has been blazing has died down place the wrapped sweet potatoes in the remaining ashes. Cover them completely with ashes and let them sit there for 30 minutes.

Use a skewer to test them and to remove them if they are tender. If not, keep them in the ashes until they are tender.

The wet newspaper feeds the flames and cooks the potatoes by light steaming.

Bracken, Onion, Carrot, Chirimen Iriko Nitsuke 179.

1 handful bracken (wild spring mountain vegetable)
3 med. onions, cut thin mawashigiri
2 carrots, cut sengiri
1 heaping Tbsp. chirimen iriko (small dried fish)
1 Tbsp. sesame oil
½ tsp. sea salt
1 Tbsp. tamari soy sauce

Gather the fresh bracken and place them in a bowl. Place one handful of wood ashes on top of them and cover with boiling water. Let this sit overnight. Wash the bracken and it is ready to cook. Bracken has too much potassium, and this method will yangize the high alkalinity.

Cut the bracken 1″ koguchigiri. Heat the oil and saute the onions. Add the chirimen iriko and saute 5 minutes. Add the bracken and saute until its color changes. Add the carrots and saute them a few minutes. Add the salt and soy sauce. Cover and cook the nitsuke until it is tender — about 10 or 15 minutes.

Daikon and Horsetail Nitsuke 180.

1 daikon, cut sengiri
1 daikon leaf, cut ¼″ koguchigiri
1 handful horsetail (clean as in 156.), cut 1″ koguchigiri
1 Tbsp. sesame oil
½ tsp. sea salt
1 Tbsp. tamari soy sauce

Heat the oil and saute the daikon leaf until it is bright green. Add the horsetail and the daikon and saute these about 10 minutes.

Add the salt and soy sauce, cover and cook the nitsuke on a medium flame until the vegetables are tender — about 10 or 15 minutes.

Deep-Fried Fish 181.

5 smelt
2 tsp. sea salt
1 Tbsp. ginger juice
1 cup whole wheat pastry flour
oil for deep-frying

Clean the fish and remove the organs. Sprinkle the salt and the ginger juice on all parts of the fish and let this sit for 10 minutes or more.

Dust the fish with whole wheat pastry flour.

Heat some deep-frying oil, then let it cool for a few minutes. Turn heat on again to medium and deep-fry fish about 7 minutes on each side until golden brown.

Strain the excess oil and serve the fish hot. This fried fish can be eaten whole, including the bones and head.

Serve with grated daikon and tamari soy sauce.

Dried Zucchini and Dried Broccoli Nitsuke 182.

1 cup dried zucchini
1 cup dried broccoli
1 Tbsp. oil
½ tsp. sea salt
1 Tbsp. tamari soy sauce

After washing vegetables, cover with water and soak them overnight. Squeeze the excess water from the vegetables.

Saute the broccoli for a few minutes, add the zucchini and saute a few minutes. Add the salt and the soy sauce. Cover and cook for 20 minutes until they are tender.

If extra water is needed for cooking, use the soaking water.

Cooked Vegetable Salad Miso Ai *(Miso Dressing)* 183.

2 bunches scallions, cut 1″ koguchigiri
2 stalks celery, cut 1″ thin sengiri (matchsticks)
1 lb. bean sprouts
2 Tbsp. lemon juice
1 heaping Tbsp. barley miso
1 heaping Tbsp. rice miso
8 cups boiling water
2 tsp. sea salt

Bring the water and salt to a boil. Add the bean sprouts and cook them for 1 minute. Remove them and let cool.

Cook the celery until the water boils, then remove and cool it. Place the scallions in this same water and cook them until they are bright green. Strain the water and let the vegetables cool. Reserve the water for soup stock.

For miso dressing: Grind both kinds of miso and the lemon juice together in a suribachi. Squeeze the excess water from the vegetables and add it to the dressing.

Mix the dressing with the vegetable salad and serve cool.

Egg Omelette 184.

1 egg
3 scallions, cut ¼″ koguchigiri
¼ tsp. sea salt
1 tsp. tamari soy sauce

Mix all the ingredients. Oil a frying pan, heat the oil and pour in the egg mixture. Cook on a medium flame until it is half done. Then turn it over and cook the other side. When it is done, fold it in half and serve hot.

Variation: For a filling inside the folded egg, use bread croutons or cooked potatoes.

Cabbage and Red Radish Pressed Salad 185.

1 small head cabbage, cut in quarters and shredded thin
1 bunch red radishes, roots cut thin koguchigiri, leaves cut thin ¼″
2 tsp. sea salt

Place the cabbage and radish leaves in a suribachi and knead with salt until they are slightly soft. Mix these thoroughly with the radish root and place this in a salad press under pressure until enough water comes from the vegetables to cover them. This should happen in a few hours.

They can be served the next day.

Hijiki Nitsuke 186.

2 cups hijiki
1 Tbsp. sesame oil
1 Tbsp. tamari soy sauce

Spread out the hijiki to remove any pieces of straw, etc., then cover with water and soak it about 20 minutes. Strain and reserve the water.

Wash the hijiki until it is free of sand and cut it in 1″ lengths. Heat the oil and saute the hijiki about 10 minutes.

Note: Strain the reserved soaking water through a fresh cotton towel before using, to remove the sediment. Taste this water. If it is too salty, use only half of it, adding plain water as necessary.

Add the soaking water to the hijiki and cook until it is tender. Add the soy sauce and cook it 10 more minutes, covered.

If there is too much liquid remaining in the pot, remove the cover and boil away the excess water.

Vegetables with Curry Sauce 187.

2 med. onions, minced
½ med. carrot, cut ichogiri
1 handful string beans, cut ¼" koguchigiri
¾ cup whole wheat pastry flour
5 cups boiling water
¼ to 1 tsp. curry powder, to taste
1 Tbsp. sea salt
1 tsp. sesame oil
2 tsp. corn oil

Heat the 2 tsp. of corn oil, add the curry powder and saute it a few minutes. Add the flour and saute it for 10 minutes on a medium flame. Set aside to cool.

Heat the 1 tsp. of sesame oil, saute the onions until they are brown, then add the string beans and saute them until the color changes. Add the carrots and saute a few minutes, then add the boiling water. Bring to a boil on a high flame, then turn the heat down to medium and cook it for 10 minutes. Add the salt and cook the vegetables 20 minutes longer or until they are tender.

Mix together the roasted flour and 2 cups of cold water. Add this to the vegetables and cook for 10 minutes. Taste and add soy sauce if necessary.

Mekabu Nitsuke 188.

1 pkg. (¾ oz.) mekabu
4 cups water
1 tsp. tamari soy sauce

Soak the mekabu in 4 cups of water. Strain and reserve soaking water.

To 1 cup soaking water add 2 cups of plain water. Add this to the mekabu and pressure-cook it for 1 hour.

When the pressure returns to normal, add soy sauce and cook it without a cover until the excess water is evaporated. Cook until it is very soft.

Mekabu is the root of wakame so it has lots of minerals. It is very tough; however, it combines well with any kind of bean soup such as lentil, pinto, kidney, etc.

Corn Bread 189.

5 cups corn meal
5 cups rice flour
10 cups unbleached white flour
2 Tbsp. corn oil
8 cups warm water
2 Tbsp. sea salt

Yeast mixture:
½ cup warm water
1 tsp. yeast
½ cup unbleached white flour

Mix the dry ingredients with the oil. Be sure and mix the oil and flour thoroughly.

Add the yeast to ½ cup warm water and allow it to sit 5 minutes. Add ½ cup flour, mix and let sit for 5 minutes until it bubbles.

Add this yeast mixture and the 8 cups of warm water to the flours, mix with a wooden spoon and let it sit overnight in a covered bowl at room temperature (or in a warm place for 4 - 5 hours).

After it has doubled in size, punch it down and let it rise again (about 1 hour). Punch down with wet hands and form into 5 large loaves. Place in pans, make a cut down the center of each loaf and place the bread in a cold oven. Bake at 450° for 1 hour.

Freshly-milled flour and meal makes the best tasting bread — like cake.

Apple - Chestnut Ring 190.

1 cup dried chestnuts
2 cups water
2 cups thinly sliced apples
1 tsp. yannoh (grain coffee)

Dough: 4 cups whole wheat pastry flour
1 tsp. sea salt
4 Tbsp. oil
1¼ cups cold water

Soak the chestnuts in water overnight, then pressure-cook them for 40 minutes. When the pressure returns to normal, mash the chestnuts until about half of them are well mashed. Let them cool and mix with the apples and yannoh.

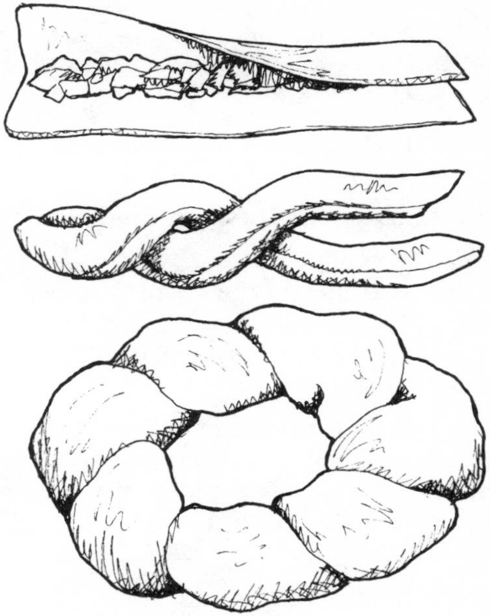

Make the dough, mixing the oil and water with the flour and salt. Knead all the ingredients well, then divide the dough in half. Roll out each half to a 5″ × 16″ rectangle. Divide the filling into 2 parts and spread it on the dough. Roll each rectangle up tightly together, form them into a ring and seal the ends.

For a nice glaze, brush egg yolk on top. Bake the ring at 450° for 30 - 40 minutes until slightly brown.

Tomato Sauce 191a.

2 medium tomatoes
2 cups onions, cut thin mawashigiri
1 Tbsp. arrowroot flour
1 tsp. sea salt
1 Tbsp. oil
2 bay leaves

Remove the skins of the tomatoes and slice them into chunks.

Heat the oil and saute the onions until they are transparent. Add the tomatoes and saute 5 minutes, then add the salt and bay leaves. Cook this sauce on a low flame for 30 minutes.

Dissolve the arrowroot flour in 3 Tbsp. of cold water, add to the tomato and onion mixture and bring to a boil. Remove the bay leaves and serve the sauce with cold somen (thin summer noodles).

Tomato Sauce with Miso 191b.

2 cups onions, cut mijingiri
½ cup pizza sauce (see 226.)
1 heaping Tbsp. barley miso
4 cups boiling water
3 bay leaves
1 Tbsp. sesame oil

Saute the onions until they are golden brown. Add the miso and saute it about 20 minutes — until it is fragrant. Add the pizza sauce and cook it for 10 minutes. Add the boiling water and bay leaves and cook the sauce for 20 - 30 minutes.

This is a very good spaghetti sauce — it is not so yin.

Lentil - Barley Soup *(Metropolitan Soup)* 192.

⅓ cup barley
⅔ cup lentils or pinto beans
2 med. onions, cut thin mawashigiri
1 carrot, cut ichogiri
½ stalk of celery, cut sainome (diced)
1 Tbsp. sesame oil
3 cups water
2 tsp. sea salt
1 tsp. tamari soy sauce

Wash the barley and soak it overnight in 1 cup of water. Wash the lentils and let them soak overnight in a separate bowl in 2 cups of water.

Cook the barley with soaking water in a pressure cooker for 15 minutes. Cook the lentils with their water in a pressure cooker until the weight begins to jiggle, then shut off the heat.

Saute the onions, celery and carrots, then add enough water to cover them. Cook 20 minutes, then add the salt, lentils and barley all at the same time. Cook the soup 30 minutes more and season with soy sauce. Add more water if necessary.

Tahini Custard 193.

1 bar kanten, diluted in 2½ cups of apple juice
1 tsp. sea salt
4 Tbsp. sweet rice flour
2 Tbsp. tahini
¼ tsp. lemon peel

Heat the diluted kanten with salt. Blend the sweet rice flour and the tahini in 2½ cups of water and add it to the hot kanten. Cook this over a medium flame, stirring occasionally, about 15 minutes.

Allow it to cool, add the lemon peel, then pour it into individual serving dishes and refrigerate it.

Serve this custard with toasted chopped almonds or apricot cream (made with dried apricots, cooked and blended) as a topping.

Amasake Cookies 194.

3 cups whole wheat pastry flour
1 cup blended amasake
½ cup warm water
½ cup sliced walnuts
¼ cup sliced raisins or whole currants
1 cup oatmeal
3 Tbsp. oil
1 tsp. sea salt

Mix the oil, salt, flour and oatmeal. In another bowl mix the amasake with warm water and add this to the dry ingredients. Also add in the fruit and nuts, mixing with a wooden spoon.

Dust a cookie sheet with oatmeal and bake the cookies at 450° until they are done.

Fresh Green Pea Rice 195.

5 cups brown rice
8 cups water
½ cup sherry or sake
2 cups fresh peas
2 tsp. sea salt

Wash the rice and soak it overnight in 8 cups of water.

Before cooking it, add the salt and liquor. Cook it covered for 20 minutes on a low flame in a heavy iron pan. Turn the flame to high for 10 minutes; steam will come out from under the cover. Turn the flame to low and cook the rice for 1 hour.

Turn off the heat and let sit for 10 minutes. Then place the fresh green peas on top of the rice and cover the pot again for 10 minutes before serving. The peas will be steam-cooked by this method.

Mix the rice thoroughly bottom to top and serve hot.

Chirashi Sushi 196.

3 cups brown rice
1 med. carrot, cut sasagaki
3 med. shiitake mushrooms, soaked 20 min., cut sengiri
3 long strips kampyo, soaked in water until soft, cut in 1″ pieces
½ cup fresh green peas
2 tsp. sea salt
4 tsp. tamari soy sauce
1 egg, beaten
½ tsp. arrowroot flour
juice of 1 lemon
1 tsp. sesame oil

Cook the rice with 4 cups of water and ½ tsp. salt under pressure for 1 hour (as in 1b.).

Saute the carrot in 1 tsp. oil. Add ¼ tsp. salt and 2 Tbsp. water to the carrot. Cover and cook until it is tender but still keeps its shape.

Reserve the soaking water from the kampyo. Strain it through cheese cloth to filter out the sediment, then bring it to a boil with the kampyo. Cook until the kampyo is transparent. If there is too much water, remove some of it. Add 2 tsp. soy sauce and continue cooking the kampyo until it is tender — about 20 minutes. Strain the excess liquid and let the kampyo cool.

Place the shiitake mushrooms back in their soaking water and boil them for 10 minutes. Add 1 tsp. soy sauce and cook 10 more minutes. Strain the excess water and let them cool.

Boil the green peas in salted water for a few minutes in an uncovered pan. Strain the water and let the peas cool.

Prepare a crepe using the beaten egg, ⅛ tsp. salt, ½ tsp. arrowroot flour and 1 tsp. water. Mix the flour and water first, then mix in the other ingredients. Oil a heavy frying pan and pour in the egg mixture. Make it very thin, almost like paper, but even. Cook until set and let cool. Cut it into 2″ long very thin strips.

Place the hot rice in a salad bowl and sprinkle with the juice of one lemon. Let it cool completely. Mix in all the ingredients thoroughly, except the egg. Use the egg as garnish.

Serve this sushi cool.

Onion Cream Miso Soup 197.

5 small whole onions
5 pieces of carrot, cut ½″ thick hasugiri
4 cups boiling water
1 heaping Tbsp. bechamel sauce (see 37.)
3 level Tbsp. barley miso
1 tsp. sesame oil

Heat the oil in a pressure cooker and saute the onions until their color changes slightly. Add the carrots and saute them for a few minutes. Add the boiling water and cook on a high flame under pressure for 5 minutes. Shut off the heat and let the pressure return to normal.

Mix the bechamel sauce with ½ cup of water and add it to the soup. Cook the soup 10 minutes more.

Soften the miso with a little of the soup stock and add it to the soup. Bring to a boil and serve immediately.

This soup is a good introduction to miso soup; it appeals to those who are just beginning macrobiotics.

Cooked Shad *(Fish)* 198.

1 whole shad, about 1 ft. long
2 cups bancha tea
7 umeboshi pits or 3 umeboshi
¼″ slice of fresh ginger

For condiment:

1 piece of ginger *or*
2″ of daikon

Remove the tail and head of the fish and cut fish into 12 pieces. Discard the tail and head. Give to dog or cat.

Mix all the ingredients together and pressure-cook them for 2 hours or until the bones are soft.

When it has cooled, serve the fish with grated ginger or grated daikon and tamari soy sauce.

The entire fish can be eaten, including the bones.

Soybean Soup 199.

2 onions, cut mawashigiri
1 burdock, cut sasagaki
1 carrot, cut sasagaki
¼ cup soybeans
½ cup water
5 cups water
1 Tbsp. chirimen iriko (optional)
1 tsp. sea salt
1 Tbsp. oil
1 Tbsp. tamari soy sauce

Soak the soybeans overnight in ½ cup of water after washing them. Then grind in a blender.

Saute the onions, burdock, chirimen iriko and then the carrot. Add the water, bring to a boil and cook for 20 minutes.

Add the salt and the soybeans. The beans will foam over, so be careful when adding them. Cook the soup 20 minutes more.

Season with soy sauce and serve it hot.

Variation: Turnip or cabbage can be substituted when burdock is out of season or is not available.

Ohsawa Corn Bread 200.

4 cups cooked brown rice
2 cups water
2 cups whole wheat flour (or pastry flour)
3 cups corn meal
½ cup buckwheat flour
1 tsp. sea salt
1 Tbsp. black or brown sesame seeds

Mix the rice and water so that all the rice grains are separate. Add the salt, all the flour and the corn meal.

Don't knead the dough; mix it gently with a wooden spoon until it is thoroughly mixed. Allow as much air as possible to get into the bread dough.

Oil a square cake pan and spread the dough over it to a 1″ thickness. Sprinkle on the sesame seeds. Using a rice paddle, make indentations in the dough so that it will be easy to break off and eat after it is baked.

Bake it in a 350° oven for 45 minutes and serve it hot.

Boiled Carrots 201.

5 carrots, cut ¼″ hasugiri
½ cup water
1 tsp. sea salt

Boil the carrots in the water in a covered pan. Cook until they are tender — almost all the water will be evaporated by that time.

Serve at once.

Bamboo Shoot Rice 202.

3 cups brown rice
3 bamboo shoots, cut rangiri
¼ cup sherry or sake
1 Tbsp. tamari soy sauce
3½ cups water

Remove the outer skins of the bamboo shoots and cut.

Soak the rice for at least 5 hours, then mix it with the sherry or sake, soy sauce and bamboo shoots. Cook under pressure as in 1b.

Strawberry and White Raisin Kanten 203.

6 cups white raisins
6 cups water
2 heaping Tbsp. kanten powder or 4 kanten bars
7 cups water
4 cups raisin puree
2 boxes of fresh strawberries
4 tsp. sea salt

Wash the strawberries in salt water and slice them.

Soak the raisins in 6 cups of water for 2 hours and cook under pressure until the pressure weight jiggles. Shut off the heat and let the pressure return to normal. Blend the raisins and their juice to a puree.

Dissolve the kanten in 7 cups of water and bring to a boil. Add the salt and cook it for 15 minutes. Stir in the raisin puree and cook 5 minutes more. Add the strawberries, stir and cook for just a few minutes.

Place in a mold to set and serve cold.

Sauteed Cabbage 204.

1 small head cabbage, cut sengiri
3 onions, cut thin mawashigiri
1 carrot, cut thin sengiri
5 green peppers, cut sengiri
2 Tbsp. sesame oil
1 tsp. sea salt

Heat the oil on a high flame. Saute the onion, then the green pepper, carrot and cabbage on a high flame until the vegetables change color.

Add the salt and saute them for a few minutes more in an uncovered pan. These vegetables will be very crisp.

Cherry Pie 205.

3 cups pitted cherries
2 cups whole wheat pastry flour
1 cup unbleached white flour
1 heaping Tbsp. arrowroot flour
3 Tbsp. cold water
3 Tbsp. oil
1 tsp. cinnamon
1 cup boiling water
1 tsp. sea salt

Mix oil, salt, flour and cinnamon, thoroughly. Add the boiling water and mix with a fork until slightly cool.

Separate this dough in two parts, to make a top and a bottom crust. Roll each out to about ¼" - ⅛" thickness.

Set the bottom crust in a lightly oiled pie pan.

Dissolve the arrowroot in cold water, mix in the cherries and place this filling in the pie shell. Cover it with the top crust and cut a cross in the center for the heat to escape.

Make your own design around the edge and bake the pie 40 minutes at 450°.

Barley - Brown Rice 206.

6 cups brown rice
4 cups barley
11 cups water
1 tsp. sea salt

Wash the grains separately. Mix them and soak them overnight.

Pressure-cook as in recipe 1b.

Barley rice is good in the summer to cool the body. In winter, use the proportions of 6 cups rice to 2 cups barley.

Cooked Salmon Head with Curry Sauce 207.

1 cup cooked salmon head
3 onions, diced
2 carrots, cut ichogiri (quarter moon)
5 small whole potatoes
1 handful snow peas
7 cups boiling water
1½ cups whole wheat pastry flour
1 Tbsp. sesame oil
½ to 1 tsp. curry powder, to taste
1 Tbsp. sea salt

Pressure cook the salmon head for 1 hour with enough water to cover it. After the pressure comes down, shred the salmon head into small pieces and cook it again for 3 hours under pressure until the bones are soft.

Heat the oil and saute the curry powder until it is slightly brown. Add the flour and cook it about 10 minutes until it is fragrant. Set aside to cool.

Boil 7 cups of water, add the onions, carrots, potatoes, cooked salmon head and 2 tsp. salt and cook until the vegetables are tender.

Make a thin batter of the flour and curry sauce mixture using cold water. Add this to the vegetables and salmon. Add salt to taste, about 1 tsp., and cook this for 20 minutes.

Five minutes before serving, add the snow peas and cook until their color changes. Serve hot.

Corn Meal 208.

1 cup corn meal
¼ tsp. sea salt
1 tsp. oil
3 - 4 cups boiling water

Saute the corn meal lightly in oil.

Over the sink, add the salt and the boiling water. Stir it well. Return to stove and cook it 30 - 45 minutes on a low flame, but keep it slightly boiling.

Bulghur 209.

3 cups bulghur
6 cups cold water
½ tsp. sea salt

Wash the bulghur and let it drain for half a day.

Roast it in a dry pan until it is fragrant. Add the water and bring to a boil. Add the salt and cook on a low flame for 1 hour.

Bulghur is a light grain, it digests fast and is good for summer meals.

Kuzu or curry sauce combine well with this grain. (See 47. and 187.).

Note: If you use boiling water, you only need to cook the bulghur 20 minutes.

Bulghur Croquettes 210.

3 cups cooked bulghur
1 med. onion, minced
½ carrot, minced
½ block tofu (squeeze out excess water using a cotton cloth)
1 Tbsp. sesame oil
2 Tbsp. corn oil
⅓ cup whole wheat pastry flour
1 tsp. sea salt
1 heaping Tbsp. minced parsley

Saute the onion until it is transparent. Add the carrot and saute it 5 minutes. Add the tofu, salt and cooked bulghur and mix thoroughly. Remove from heat and let the mixture cool to body temperature. Mix in the pastry flour.

Make patties about 1″ thick. Heat a frying pan, add 2 Tbsp. oil and place the patties in the pan. Cover and cook them for 7 minutes on each side over a medium flame.

Use the leftover oil in the pan to make a bechamel sauce (as in 37.). Cover the croquettes with bechamel sauce and the minced parsley.

Cherry Kanten 211.

4 cups apple juice
2 cups water
2½ bars kanten
1 cup pitted cherries
1 tsp. sea salt

Wash the kanten and soak it in water for 20 minutes.

Bring it to a boil with the salt, uncovered, and cook for 15 minutes. Add the cherries and boil it again. Add the apple juice and cook it a few minutes more, stirring frequently.

Place it in a mold and let it cool. Place in refrigerator. Serve cold.

Creamed Cabbage 212.

½ head of cabbage, cut into 1″ squares
¼ cup whole wheat pastry flour
2 cups water
½ tsp. sea salt
1 tsp. tamari soy sauce (to taste)

Saute the flour in oil. (We used the last tempura pot, which was still quite oily, to saute this flour today.) Roast it until it has a fragrant, nut-like smell. Remove it from the pan and let it cool.

In another pot, bring 1 cup of water to a boil and add the salt and cabbage. Cover and cook the cabbage until it is tender.

Mix 1 cup of water with the roasted flour and add this to the cooked cabbage. Stir this, bring it to a boil and cook it on a low flame for 5 minutes.

If more salt is needed, add soy sauce to taste.

Collard Green, Broccoli and Sweet Potato Nitsuke 213.

1 bunch collard greens, cut 1″ koguchigiri
2 stalks broccoli - separate flowers, cut stems ¼″ koguchigiri
3 med. sweet potatoes, cut into 1″ cubes
1 Tbsp. sesame oil
½ tsp. sea salt
1 Tbsp. tamari soy sauce

Saute the broccoli stems. After the color changes, add the collard greens and the broccoli flowers. When the color becomes bright green, add the sweet potatoes and saute them until they are slightly transparent.

Add the salt and soy sauce, cover and add water if necessary. Cook it until all the vegetables are tender (about 30 minutes).

Rice Salad 214.

3 cups cooked brown rice
2 stalks celery, cut thin hasugiri
½ head of lettuce, cut sengiri
2 cucumbers, cut thin koguchigiri
1 tomato (optional)

Umeboshi Dressing:

2 salt plums
1 Tbsp. shiso leaves, sliced thin
1 Tbsp. oil
1 minced onion
½ tsp. grated orange rind

Cut all the vegetables very thin.

Remove the pits from the salt plums and grind plums in

a suribachi with the shiso leaves. Add the oil, grind them again, then add the onion. Let the dressing sit for 20 minutes.

Add the orange rind and the vegetables to the dressing. Mix thoroughly and add the rice.

If the rice is very dry, sprinkle a little water on it before mixing it with the vegetables.

Raisin Buns with Strawberry Topping 215a.

3 cups whole wheat pastry flour
3 cups unbleached white flour
½ cup raisins or currants
½ tsp. yeast
½ cup warm water
1 Tbsp. oil
1 tsp. sea salt
3 cups warm water
2 heaping Tbsp. white flour

Mix the yeast with ½ cup warm water and let it sit for 5 minutes. Add the 2 Tbsp. of white flour and let this sit until the mixture bubbles.

In a large bowl, combine the flours and this yeast mixture. In a separate bowl, mix the oil, salt and 3 cups of warm water. (Use part of this water to wash out the yeast mixture.) Add this to the flour mixture. Add the raisins, mix all ingredients together thoroughly and let the dough sit for 4 hours in a warm place — until it doubles in size.

Punch it down and let it rise again.

Dust a cake pan with corn meal. Wet your hand and make balls from the dough, 1½" in diameter. Place them close together in the pan. Place in a cold oven, turn it on to 450° and bake the buns for 45 - 50 minutes, until they turn slightly brown.

Strawberry Topping:

4 boxes of fresh strawberries
3 cups apple butter
2 cups boiling water
1 tsp. sea salt
2 heaping Tbsp. arrowroot
2 tsp. vanilla extract

Wash the strawberries and cut them into quarters.

Mix the apple butter, salt and boiling water and bring it to a boil. Add the strawberries and bring to a boil again.

Dissolve the arrowroot in ¼ cup of cold water and add it to the mixture. Bring this to a boil. When the mixture thickens, set it aside to cool. Add the vanilla when the mixture has cooled slightly, and serve the topping over the buns.

Strawberry Delight 215b.

3 boxes of fresh strawberries, sliced
2 cups apple juice
1 tsp. sea salt
2 heaping Tbsp. arrowroot flour

Dissolve the arrowroot in ¼ cup of cold water. Mix the apple juice with the strawberries and bring this to a boil on a high flame. Add the arrowroot, bring to a boil again and let it cool.

This is very delicious, much like strawberry jello.

Zucchini Squash and Onion Nitsuke 216.

7 med. zucchini squash, cut ¼″ wagiri
3 med. onions, cut ¼″ mawashigiri
2 tsp. sesame oil
¼ tsp. sea salt
2 tsp. tamari soy sauce

Heat the oil and saute the onions until they are transparent. Add the squash and saute it a few minutes. Cover and cook on a medium flame. After 5 minutes of cooking, stir the vegetables; then stir again in 5 more minutes. Add the salt and soy sauce. Continue cooking on a low flame for 10 minutes or until it is tender.

Remove the cover and cook on a high flame for a few minutes to evaporate some of the extra liquid.

Cucumber Salad 217.

3 cucumbers - peel them if the skins are waxed
2 tsp. sea salt
3 Tbsp. lemon juice

Remove the head of the cucumber, dip it in salt and replace it on the cucumber. Rub this around the cut end to take out the bitterness. Then cut the cucumber in very thin slices (koguchigiri). Sprinkle on the salt and let it sit for 10 minutes.

When the water comes out of the cucumbers, they will be soft and you can squeeze out any excess water. Then mix with lemon juice and serve about 5 minutes later.

Variation: Instead of lemon juice, substitute 3 Tbsp. rice vinegar or 3 Tbsp. equal amounts of lemon and orange juice.

Cold Salmon with Gravy 218.

5 pieces of fresh salmon
2 med. onions, cut mijingiri
2″ piece of carrot, cut mijingiri
1 tsp. sesame oil
1 Tbsp. ginger juice
1 tsp. sea salt
¼ cup boiling water

Gravy: ¼ cup whole wheat pastry flour
2 tsp. corn oil
1 tsp. sea salt
½ cup cold water

Sprinkle the ginger juice and 1 tsp. salt on both sides of the salmon and let it sit for 20 minutes.

Heat 1 tsp. of sesame oil, saute the onions and carrots and place the salmon on top of the vegetables. Add ¼ cup of boiling water around the edge of the pan. Cover and cook on a medium flame for 20 minutes. Set it aside to cool.

Heat 2 tsp. of corn oil and saute ¼ cup of pastry flour until it is fragrant. Set it aside to cool, then mix the flour with ½ cup of cold water.

After the salmon is completely cool, remove it and place it on a plate. Add the flour and water mixture to the onions and carrots and bring this to a boil. If necessary add more water, with 1 tsp. salt. Cook on a low flame for 20 minutes.

Pour the gravy on top of the salmon and serve it immediately.

Sauteed Onion and Potato with Salmon and Egg 219.

3 potatoes, cut sengiri
5 onions, cut thin mawashigiri
2 eggs, beaten
½ cup baked salmon, shredded
2 Tbsp. oil
2 tsp. sea salt

Heat the oil and saute the potatoes in a covered pan until they are half done. Add the onions and saute them until they are transparent. Sprinkle with salt, cover and cook the vegetables until they are tender.

Mix the egg with the salmon. Cover the vegetables with this mixture but don't stir it. Let it cook in a covered pan until the egg is firm.

Serve it hot.

Tofu, Snow Peas and White Rice Miso Soup 220.

¼ block tofu, cut ½″ sainome (diced)
5 cups boiling water
10 snow peas
2 heaping Tbsp. white rice miso

Bring the water to a boil, add the snow peas and cook for 5 minutes without a cover. Add the tofu and bring the soup to a boil. Shut off the heat, add the miso and serve it hot.

Hijiki - Carrot Nitsuke 221.

1 cup hijiki, cut in 1″ lengths
1 med. carrot, cut sengiri
2 tsp. sesame oil
½ tsp. tamari soy sauce

Remove the dried straw and dirt from the hijiki and soak it for 10 minutes in enough water to cover it. Drain and reserve the water. Strain this water through a cotton cloth and use it for cooking. Rinse the hijiki 2 or 3 times by placing it in a container full of water. Then strain and cut it.

Heat the oil and saute the carrot until it is slightly soft. Add the hijiki and saute it for 5 minutes. Then add the reserved soaking water. Bring this to a boil on a high flame, turn flame to medium and cook until the hijiki is tender — 30 to 45 minutes.

Add the soy sauce and cook 5 minutes more. If there is too much liquid, remove the cover and let some of it boil away.

Variation: 2 onions, cut thin mawashigiri
½ cup burdock, cut sasagaki

The above vegetables can be substituted for the carrot.

Somen 222.

1 lb. somen
8 cups water
clear soup (see 16.) or tomato
sauce (see 191a.)

Bring the water to a boil and add the somen, stirring it with chopsticks to keep the noodles separated. Cover the pot. Bring to a boil, then shut off the flame. Drain the water and wash the noodles in cold water until they are completely cold.

Serve them immediately with clear soup or tomato sauce.

If you plan to serve the somen later, use this method to keep them from sticking together: pick up a serving with your fingers, twist the noodles and place them in a serving bowl. Repeat this until all the somen is in the bowl.

Sesame Balls 223.

- 1 cup sesame seeds, roasted
- ½ tsp. grated lemon rind
- 1 Tbsp. carob (powder)
- 1 tsp. sesame oil, heated and cooled

Grind the sesame seeds, add oil and mix all the ingredients together. Add water by drops until there is enough moisture to form a nice ball about 1″ in diameter.

Variation: If you like sweet sesame balls, use yinnie syrup to make moisture instead of the water.

Wakame Cucumber Salad 224.

- ½ cup dried wakame
- 3 cucumbers, cut thin koguchigiri
- 2 tsp. sea salt
- 3 Tbsp. rice vinegar *or* 2 Tbsp. lemon juice *or* 3 Tbsp. orange juice

Soak the wakame in enough water to cover it for about 10 minutes, until it is soft. Strain and reserve the water for soup stock. Then cut it in 1″ strips.

Mix the cucumber with 1 tsp. salt and let it sit for 10 minutes. Then squeeze out the excess water.

Mix the remaining salt with the vinegar (or lemon or orange juice). Mix this in with the wakame and the cucumber. Let sit 10 - 20 minutes and serve the salad cold.

Each time you serve it, mix it again first.

French Bread Pudding 225.

- 1 loaf whole wheat French bread, hard and old
- 2 cups water
- ⅓ cup raisins, sliced thinly
- 2 bananas, cut into ¼″ strips
- 1 egg, beaten

Slice bread into 1″ pieces and tear it into bits. Mix all ingredients and let them sit for 20 minutes, or until bread is soft. Add more water if necessary.

Place this in a baking dish and pat it down. Bake it at 450° for 45 minutes or until it is slightly brown.

It can be served hot or cold.

For variety, use fruits that are in season. In winter, 1 heaping Tbsp. of grated cheese can be added and milk can be used instead of water.

Tomato - Cheese or Salmon Pizza 226a.

Dough:
- 3 cups unbleached white flour
- 1 tsp. yeast
- 1 cup warm water
- 2 heaping Tbsp. unbleached white flour
- 1 tsp. sea salt

Covering:
- 4 heaping Tbsp. tomato sauce (7 med. tomatoes)
- 3 tsp. minced parsley
- 2 heaping Tbsp. salmon, flaked (home-made canned salmon) *or* 4 heaping Tbsp. grated cheese (raw milk cheese)

Dip the tomatoes in boiling water for a few minutes, then let them drain and cool. Peel off their skins and chop them into small pieces. Bring them to a boil uncovered in a sauce pan and cook on a low flame 4 - 5 hours, or until the tomatoes become like a sauce.

Dissolve the yeast in ½ cup of warm water. Add 2 heaping Tbsp. white flour and set this in a warm place until it bubbles.

Mix 3 cups of flour with the yeast mixture. Add ½ cup warm water and the salt and knead this dough to an ear lobe consistency. Add more flour if necessary. Cover the bowl and let the dough sit in a warm area.

After 1 hour, punch it down. Let it rise again for 30 minutes.

Punch it down again and separate it into 4 portions. Roll out each portion on a floured table or cutting board. Place in pizza pans.

Mix the parsley and the tomato sauce and spread this on the dough. Sprinkle on the cheese or the salmon and bake the pizzas at 400° for 20 minutes. Serve them hot from the oven.

Vegetable Pizza *(Variation)* 226b.

Dough:
- 4 cups whole wheat flour
- 3 cups unbleached white flour
- 1 tsp. sea salt
- 2½ cups warm water
- 1 tsp. yeast
- 2 Tbsp. corn oil

Covering:
- 1 pkg. (12 oz.) fresh mushrooms, cut thin koguchigiri
- 3 small green peppers, cut thin koguchigiri (same size as mushrooms)
- 3 small onions, cut thin mawashigiri
- 6 small tomatoes, cut thin, same size as mushrooms
- ½ tsp. sea salt
- 1 pkg. raw milk cheese (1 lb.)

Make the pizza dough the same as in 226a.

Slice each vegetable and mix with ½ tsp. salt. Spread on the pizza dough in this order: green pepper, onion, mushroom and tomato.

Sprinkle grated cheese on top. Bake the same as 226a.

This recipe makes 3 large cookie sheet size pizzas — about 13″ × 19″ cookie sheet size.

String Bean - Celery Nitsuke with Sesame Butter 227a.

25 med. string beans, whole
3 stalks celery, cut ¼″ hasugiri
1 heaping Tbsp. sesame butter
½ tsp. sea salt
1 Tbsp. tamari soy sauce
½ cup boiling water

Bring the water to a boil, add the string beans with the salt and cook on a medium flame for 10 minutes. Add the celery and cook 5 minutes longer, stirring occasionally. Add the sesame butter to the vegetables and continue stirring for 5 minutes.

Add the soy sauce to taste and cook a few more minutes.

String Bean, Onion, Carrot Nitsuke 227b.

1 handful string beans, cut hasugiri in half
2 med. onions, cut ¼″ mawashigiri
1 small carrot, cut sasagaki
2 tsp. sesame oil
¼ tsp. sea salt
1 - 2 tsp. tamari soy sauce

Heat the oil and saute the onions until they are transparent. Add the string beans and cook them in a covered pot until they are bright green. Add the carrots and saute them a few minutes, then add the salt and soy sauce. Cook the nitsuke on a low flame for 10 minutes, or until juice comes from the vegetables.

Raise the flame to medium and cook the vegetables until they are tender. Turn off the heat and sprinkle on soy sauce, to taste.

Serve at once.

Apple Butter made from Dried Apples 228.

4 cups dried apples

Soak the apples with sufficient water to cover them for 30 minutes. Cook them under pressure for 20 minutes. When the pressure comes down to normal, stir the apples thoroughly.

Serve this hot or cold.

This is very sweet apple butter.

Cucumber with Miso 229.

1 fresh cold cucumber
1 tsp. barley miso
sea salt

Cut ¼″ off the stem end of the cucumber. Rub both cut ends with salt until they become juicy.

Wash the cucumber and slice it into ¼″ wagiri. Serve slices with miso topping.

If you are not using an organic cucumber, peel off all the skin.

This is good for a summer snack or appetizer. It is very refreshing.

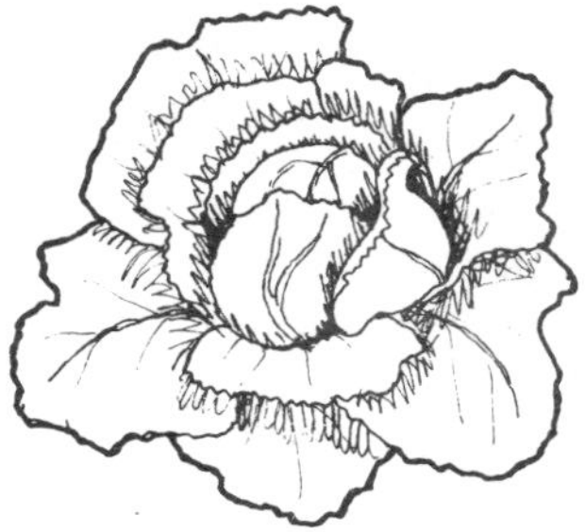

Sour Cabbage 230.

2 med. cabbage
1 Tbsp. sea salt
5 bay leaves
Japanese (or other) salad press

Quarter the cabbages. Wash and drain them ½ a day.

Core them and slice as thinly as possible. Place 2 handfuls of cabbage in a suribachi or bowl and add ½ tsp. of salt. Knead the cabbage gently until it begins to soften. Prepare all the cabbage with the salt in this way, 2 handfuls at a time. Save the cores for cooking.

Place cabbage in the salad press, about 3 handfuls at a time, along with 2 bay leaves. Press this strongly at room temperature for a couple of days, or until a white bubbly fermentation appears. Remove and press remainder of cabbage in this manner.

Pressed cabbage can be packed tightly in a glass jar, or it can be kept in the salad press under a very light pressure. Store in the refrigerator.

You can serve this up to 5 weeks or so.

Instant Cabbage and Cucumber Pressed Salad 231.

1 med. cabbage, cut sengiri
2 med. cucumbers, cut koguchigiri
2 tsp. sea salt

Put the cabbage and salt in a suribachi and rub it hard. Squeeze the excess juice from the cabbage. Mix in the cucumber. Chill before serving. If this salad is too salty, rinse it with cold water in a strainer.

Variation: Before squeezing the cabbage, mix in the cucumber and press the salad in a salad press. Serve 8 - 24 hours later, after chilling it.

Dill Pickles 232.

50 pickling cucumbers
3 stalks dill
12 bay leaves
1 clove garlic
½ cup sea salt
3 qts. water
2 onions, quartered

Wash, drain and dry the cucumbers. Place them in layers standing up in a large jar or crock — 1 row of cucumbers, then the blossom ends of dill. Add the onions, a bit of garlic and 2 bay leaves at the top of each layer. Repeat this until the jar is full.

Boil the salt and the water until all the salt is dissolved. Let it cool. Pour this over the pickles and let them stand in a room for a few days. Skim the scum from the top.

Place the pickles under refrigeration after a few days.

Fresh Corn Tortillas with Scallion and Oily Miso 233.

3 cobs fresh corn
2 cups whole wheat flour
15 scallions, white part only
⅓ cup barley miso
6 Tbsp. sesame oil
½ tsp. sea salt

Remove the corn husks and slice the kernels off the cob with a knife. Rub off the remaining parts of the kernels with the back of the knife. Grind the kernels in a blender. Add the flour and the salt and knead this into a stiff dough of ear lobe consistency.

Roll this into tortillas ¼″ thick and with a 4″ diameter.

Heat a frying pan, add sesame oil and fry the tortillas until both sides are golden brown. Keep them in the oven in a covered dish.

Cut the whites of scallions 2″ long sengiri style and soak them in cold water until they become crispy and cold. Then drain off the water.

Grind the miso in a suribachi. Heat up a pan, add 4 Tbsp. of sesame oil and the ground miso and saute until a fragrant smell arises.

Serve miso to each person in small bowls. Tortillas can be arranged on a large serving plate with the scallions in the middle. Each person should put one tortilla on his plate, add the scallions and miso and then roll up the tortilla with the filling. Eat them with your fingers, a fork or chopsticks.

These are really good as a summer food. You can substitute them for rice at dinner or use them as an afternoon snack.

Tostadas 234.

2 cups cooked rice
2 cups cooked pinto or kidney beans (see 32.)
1 head lettuce, cut thin sengiri (shredded)
3 Tbsp. tahini or sesame butter
4 - 6 Tbsp. tamari soy sauce
corn tortillas
1 bunch scallions, chopped
1 box cherry tomatoes

Cook the rice and beans as usual — the beans should be creamy, not dry.

Make a tahini/tamari sauce: add water to tahini until it is the consistency of cream. Add the soy sauce to taste. Bring this almost to a boil, stirring constantly. It will thicken.

Deep-fry or pan-fry the tortillas until they are crisp. You can make your own tortillas (see 233.).

To assemble the tostada, lay a tortilla on a plate. Cover it with rice, then a layer of beans. Sprinkle on shredded lettuce and pour the tahini sauce over it. Sprinkle with scallions and garnish with ½ cherry tomato or a small wedge of regular tomato.

It is best if the tortilla, rice, beans and sauce are piping hot and the lettuce and scallions are crispy and cold. Serve immediately.

Cold Somen or Udon with Clear Soup 235.

Somen (222.) *or* Udon (53.)
1 cucumber, cut thin koguchigiri
½ bunch scallions
5 - 7 cherry tomatoes
3 red radishes, cut in flower shape
Clear soup (see 16.)

Chill the somen or udon by placing it in a large glass bowl with ice water. Slice a few pieces of cucumber, radish, tomato and green scallions (cut scallion in long strips) as a garnish and float them on top of the noodles with ice cubes.

Allow the soup to cool but don't refrigerate it. Garnish with scallions (see 16b.) or grated ginger.

Serve the chilled noodles and vegetables in the large bowl with ice in the center of the table. Each person can combine the cooled soup with some noodles. This is an excellent summer dish.

Toasted Rice Balls with Soy Sauce or Miso 236.

cooked brown rice
miso or tamari

Make rice balls with fresh or slightly spoiled rice (see 125.). Toast the rice balls on top of the stove on a Japanese toaster, or in the oven.

Toast both sides at 350° until they are crispy. Brush them with tamari soy sauce or spread miso on them. Then toast them again for a few minutes.

This is a good appetizer.

Umeboshi Pit Juice 237.

1 cup umeboshi pits

Place the pits into a porcelain pan and cover with water, about ½" above the pits. Bring them to a boil on a high flame, then turn flame down to low and continue to boil on a low flame, covered, for 1 hour.

Strain and reserve the juice and throw away the pits. Keep the juice in a glass jar at room temperature.

This is a very good salad dressing or, mixed with cool water, it makes a very good summer drink. It is very refreshing.

Thousand Island Salad Dressing 238.

1 med. onion, minced
½ stalk celery, cut small
1 apple, cored and cut small
2 Tbsp. oil (cooked and cold)
⅓ cup umeboshi pit juice (see 237.)

Blend all the ingredients in a blender and keep it cold.

Variation: Any left-over fresh vegetables can be used.

Note: If you don't have umeboshi pit juice, you can use 1 tsp. of Plum Extract diluted in ⅓ cup of water with 1 tsp. sea salt and 1 tsp. tamari soy sauce. If necessary, add more salt or Plum Extract.

Bean Salad

239.

1 cup pinto, kidney or Northern white beans
1 head lettuce, cut into ¼" sengiri
3 stalks celery, cut thin koguchigiri
1 cucumber, cut thin koguchigiri
2 small onions, cut thin mawashigiri
⅓ cup umeboshi pit juice *or* ¼ cup rice vinegar *or* 3 Tbsp. lemon juice
1 heaping Tbsp. minced onions
2 Tbsp. used oil
2 tsp. sea salt

Soak the beans 4 - 5 hours, then bring them to a boil on a high flame with 1 tsp. salt. Reduce the heat to low and continue to cook them 45 minutes or until they are tender. If necessary, add more water. Drain and cool the beans.

Mix the oil, umeboshi juice (or vinegar or lemon juice) and 1 tsp. salt together until the oil gets dark. Mix in the minced onions and let the dressing sit for 20 minutes.

Mix this with the beans first, then toss in the remaining vegetables. If necessary, add more salt.

Note: When George Ohsawa came to Chico in the fall of 1964, he was surprised by the warm climate. Thus, he recommended that beans could be eaten often, as in the Mexican diet. However, Ohsawa also suggested that lots of spice or hot sauce should not be used often. I believe that hot sauce and spice tend to make one nervous and weaken the brain. They are also very bad for those who have hemmorhoids.

In a hot season one should eat less brown rice, substituting bulghur, barley, fresh corn or corn meal, noodles and also more beans and vegetables.

Summer Vegetable Macaroni Soup

240.

2 med. onions, cut thin mawashigiri
3 scallions, cut ¼" koguchigiri
1 stalk celery, cut thin hasugiri
1 small tomato, boiled, skinned and cut ¼" sainome
2 - 3 cups whole wheat macaroni
2 tsp. sesame oil
8 cups boiling water
1 Tbsp. tamari soy sauce
3 bay leaves (optional)
2 - 3 ears of corn
½ tsp. sea salt

Cut the corn off the cob slicing downward in sections. Cut each section 3 times, then with the back of the knife scrape off the remaining kernels.

Place the tomato in a pan of boiling water for 1 minute. Cool and peel off the skin. Slice the whole tomato sainome.

Wash the macaroni in cold water and let it drain.

Heat the oil and saute the onions until they are transparent. Add the tomato, saute it 5 minutes. Add the corn and celery and saute a few minutes until the celery turns bright green. Add the boiling water and bring to a boil. Add a bay leaf and the macaroni. Cover and bring to a boil again, then lower the flame and cook for 20 minutes.

Add the salt and continue cooking until the macaroni is tender. Then mix in scallions and soy sauce to taste. Serve immediately.

Use a larger amount of macaroni to make this soup thicker if you wish.

Note: Tomatoes are not good for sick people. For them, substitute cabbage leaves.

Corn on the Cob 241a.

5 ears of fresh corn
½ cup boiling water
2 tsp. sea salt

Place the water in a pressure cooker with a steamer rack. Add the corn and sprinkle it with salt. Cook it on a high flame until the pressure top jiggles. Turn the flame to medium for 7 minutes, then turn it off. Remove the lid when the pressure returns to normal and serve hot.

Corn on the Cob *(Outdoor Cooking)* 241b.

5 ears of fresh corn
2 tsp. sea salt
water

Place the corn in the pot and add enough water to cover about 2-3″ above the corn. Add the salt and bring to a boil on a high fire. Rotate the corn from top to bottom and bring it to a boil again. Remove it from the pot when tender and serve hot.

You can sprinkle on more salt if desired.

Leftover water from cooking corn can be used for soup stock, stews and kuzu sauce.

Note: Corn is good for the kidneys. Eating too much corn can cause diarrhea. Raw corn can cause skin abscesses.

Top of Stove Bread *(Wood Stove)* 242.

10 cups whole wheat flour
5 cups rice flour
5 cups warm water
4 tsp. sea salt
2 tsp. corn oil

Mix the flours together. In a separate bowl mix the water, salt and oil and add this to the flour. Knead ingredients together until the dough is the consistency of an ear lobe.

Separate it into 4 loaves and wrap each loaf twice with aluminum foil, folding in the ends.

Cook them in a wood stove, placing the loaves on an iron sheet for 2 hours. Cook the bottom for 20 minutes, then turn them over and cook the top for 20 minutes. Place each loaf on its side and cook for 20 minutes, then cook the opposite side for 20 minutes. Cook the top and bottom again for 20 minutes each.

Note: Any combination of flours can be substituted. Cooked grains can also be added.

Pear Butter 243.

Core some pears and slice them thinly. Place the cut pears in an iron or heavy stainless steel pot and cook them for 1 hour on a low flame.

When the natural juices appear, stir the pears and cook them until they are tender, on a medium flame. If they are watery, remove the cover and let some of the juice evaporate to suit your taste.

Barley Miso Soup 244.

⅓ cup barley
2 med. onions, cut thin mawashigiri
2 med. carrots, cut thin sengiri
½ stalk celery, cut thin hasugiri
1 tsp. sesame oil
1 heaping Tbsp. barley miso
5 cups boiling water

Wash and soak the barley in ⅔ cup of cold water overnight or at least 5 hours. Cook it in a pressure cooker for 20 minutes, or cook it in a regular pot (with extra water) 1½ hours or until the barley is tender.

Heat the oil and saute the onions until they are transparent. Add the carrots and saute them a few minutes. Then saute the celery until its color changes.

Add the boiling water and bring the soup to a boil on a high flame. Add the barley. Be sure to separate it so it does not remain in a large lump. Cook the soup 45 minutes to 1 hour on a low flame, adding more water if necessary.

Dilute the miso with some liquid from the soup and mix it into the soup. Serve immediately.

Tekka 245.

1 med. burdock root
1½″ of lotus root
½″ of carrot
1 tsp. grated ginger
5 chirimen iriko (dried fish), optional
1½ cups hacho or mugi miso
½ cup sesame oil to taste

Mince all the vegetables separately. Cut very fine.

Heat the oil in a wok and saute the burdock until its bitter smell is gone. Add the iriko, lotus root and carrot, in that order. Add the ginger and saute it well.

Add the miso and mix it thoroughly with the vegetables. Cook this 3 - 4 hours over a low flame until it is dry and crumbly.

Store in a jar and use as a condiment.

Polenta Potage 246.

2 med. onions, cut ¼″ mawashigiri
2 med. carrots, cut ¼″ ichogiri
2 ears of fresh corn (see 233.)
1 small tomato, cut ¼″ sainome (diced)
½ cup corn meal
1 Tbsp. sesame oil
2 tsp. sea salt
8 cups boiling water

Heat 1 tsp. of oil and roast the corn meal for about 7 minutes. Remove it from the pan.

Heat 2 tsp. of oil and saute the onions until they are transparent. Add the tomato and saute it for 5 minutes. Add the carrots and saute a few minutes. Next add the corn and saute.

Add the boiling water, bring all this to a boil and then add the corn meal. Cook this for 1 hour on a low flame, adding extra water if necessary.

Add the salt and serve in 20 minutes.

Note: You can use already-cooked corn meal in this recipe and cut down the cooking time.

Cabbage with Kuzu Sauce 247.

1 head cabbage, cut into 1″ squares
½ cup leftover dried daikon
  nitsuke (optional)
½ tsp. sea salt
2 tsp. tamari soy sauce
1 Tbsp. arrowroot or kuzu powder
boiling water

Heat the oil and saute the cabbage until its color changes to bright green. Cover it with boiling water and add salt. Cook for 20 minutes on medium flame.

Then add the leftover daikon nitsuke and soy sauce to taste. Dissolve the kuzu in 3 Tbsp. of cold water and add it to the cabbage. Cook this until it makes a thick sauce.

Clear Soup with Cucumber 248.

1 cucumber, cut 1″ wagiri
3″ × 4″ piece of dashi kombu
½ tsp. sea salt
1 tsp. tamari soy sauce
5 cups water

Place the kombu in cold water and bring it to a boil on a low flame. Boil it about 30 minutes, then take kombu out and reserve for nitsuke.

Add the cucumber and salt to the soup stock and cook for 30 minutes or until the cucumber is tender.

Add the soy sauce and serve each person a piece of cucumber with the soup.

Apple - Pear Kanten 249.

1½ bars kanten
2 cups water
1 cup apple butter (see 152.)
1 cup sliced pears, bite-size
1 tsp. sea salt

Wash and soak the kanten in cold water for 20 minutes, then bring it to a boil and add the salt. Cook for 20 minutes in an uncovered pot.

Add the apple butter and the pears and bring it to a boil again. Stir and cook this 5 more minutes.

Rinse the kanten mold or bowl with cold water. Pour in the kanten mixture and let it cool and harden before serving.

Azuki Hoto *(Azuki with Home-Made Noodles)* 250.

1 cup azuki beans
3 cups water
1 med. turnip, cut into bite-size pieces
1 med. onion, cut thin mawashigiri
5 Chinese cabbage leaves, cut into
  1″ squares
½ med. carrot, cut sengiri
1 Tbsp. sesame oil
2 - 3 tsp. sea salt
8 cups boiling water

Noodle dough: 2 cups whole wheat flour
⅔ cup boiling water
½ tsp. sea salt

Wash the azuki beans and soak them in 1½ cups of water for 5 hours.

Bring them to a boil and add ½ cup of water. Repeat this two more times. Cook the beans on medium heat until they are tender (about 1 hour).

Note: Do not pressure-cook the azuki beans; they will taste bitter.

For noodles: Mix the flour, boiling water and salt. Cover this with a clean cloth and then a straw mat, and step on it to knead it — about 10 or 15 minutes. Sprinkle a board with flour and roll out the dough until it is ¼″ thick. Sprinkle flour on the dough, fold it in half; sprinkle flour on this and fold again. Repeat this until the dough is 2″ wide. Cut this into ¼″ horizontal strips. Uncooked noodles should look like an accordion.

Heat the oil and saute the onions, turnips, cabbage and carrots. Add the 8 cups of boiling water and cook the vegetables until they are tender. Add the salt, the azuki beans and the home-made noodles. Cook this 10 - 20 minutes more, until the noodles are soft. Serve immediately.

Pan-Fried Eggplant with Lemon Miso Sauce

5 small eggplants, cut in halves
3 Tbsp. sesame oil
3 Tbsp. barley miso
½ tsp. lemon rind, grated
1 tsp. lemon juice

Cut a grille design into each piece of eggplant on the round side, somewhat resembling basket-weaving (see *kikko* cutting style).

Heat 2 tsp. of oil, place a layer of eggplant in a covered frying pan and cook it on a medium flame for 5 minutes. Adding more oil if necessary, turn and cook the eggplant for a few minutes until each piece is tender. Serve the cut side up with the sauce covering.

Lemon miso sauce: Heat 1 tsp. of oil and saute the miso until it is fragrant. Add 5 Tbsp. of water and bring to a boil. Then turn off the heat. Add the lemon rind and let it cool. Mix in the lemon juice and serve the sauce.

Variation: Oily Miso Sauce

2 - 3 tsp. sesame oil
1 Tbsp. barley miso
½ cup water

Saute the miso until it has a fragrant smell. Add the water and bring it to a boil.

Oily miso is good for any cooked grain or for steamed vegetables.

Noodle Gratin 252.

8 cups leftover fried noodles (see 29.)

Bechamel Sauce:

1 cup whole wheat pastry flour
1 Tbsp. oil
4 - 5 cups water
1 - 2 tsp. sea salt

For sauce preparation, see recipe 37. The ingredients differ here to allow for flavor in the fried noodles.

Mix ⅓ of the sauce with the noodles and place in a casserole dish. Press them down and pour the remainder of the sauce over the noodles.

Bake the gratin at 450° for 30 minutes or until it bubbles.

Togan or Cucumber with Kuzu Sauce 253.

3″ diameter, 5″ long piece of togan (Chinese cucumber squash) *or* 2 cucumbers, peeled and cut in 1″ wagiri
2 med. shiitake mushrooms, soaked 20 min. in warm water, then cut sengiri
2 heaping tsp. kuzu or arrowroot, dissolved in ½ cup cold water
2 heaping tsp. sesame oil
3 cups boiling water
½ tsp. sea salt
1 Tbsp. tamari soy sauce
1 heaping Tbsp. parsley, chopped

Cut the togan in half, remove the seeds and peel the skin. Cut into quarters, then slice 1″ thick.

Heat the oil and saute the mushrooms a few minutes. Add the togan or cucumber and saute until it is transparent. Add the soaking water from the mushrooms, the salt and the boiling water and cook the vegetables for 20 minutes or until they are tender.

Add the dissolved kuzu and bring it to a boil. Add the soy sauce and boil it again.

Serve this immediately, with chopped parsley for decoration.

Carrot, Carrot-Top and Fresh Corn Nitsuke 254.

2 med. carrots, cut sengiri
2 carrot-tops, cut ¼″ koguchigiri
1 med. ear of corn
2 tsp. sesame oil
¼ tsp. sea salt
1 Tbsp. tamari soy sauce

Remove kernels from corn with a knife.

Heat the oil and saute the carrot-tops until the color changes to bright green. Add the corn and the carrot, sauteeing each for 5 minutes. Sprinkle on the salt and soy sauce. Mix and cover the vegetables. Cook them on a low flame for 10 minutes.

When juice from the vegetables appears, increase the heat to medium and cook it for 10 minutes. Stir, let it cook 5 more minutes and serve.

Banana Squash, String Bean and Onion Nitsuke 255.

5″ diameter, 5″ long piece of banana squash, cut 1″ square
2 med. onions, cut thin mawashigiri
10 string beans, cut in 1½″ lengths
1 Tbsp. sesame oil
¼ tsp. sea salt
1½ Tbsp. tamari soy sauce

Heat the oil and saute the onions until they are transparent. Add the string beans and the squash. Saute each vegetable 5 minutes. Sprinkle with salt and soy sauce and cook in a covered pan on a low flame for 10 minutes.

After the juice comes out of the vegetables, cook them on a medium flame for 20 minutes.

Shut off the flame before the squash is completely cooked.

Note: If no water has appeared after the first 10 minutes of cooking, add ⅓ cup of boiling water around the edge of the pan.

Cabbage, Bean Sprouts and Carrot Nitsuke 256.

½ small head cabbage, cut sengiri
1 carrot, cut sengiri
2 cups bean sprouts
1 Tbsp. oil
½ tsp. sea salt

Heat 1 tsp. of oil and saute the bean sprouts on a high flame for a few minutes until they become slightly transparent. Then remove and set them aside to cool.

Heat 2 tsp. of oil and saute the cabbage and then the carrots. When the cabbage becomes transparent, sprinkle with salt and saute a few minutes longer. Then add the bean sprouts and mix well.

Serve when the bean sprouts are heated. Tamari soy sauce may be added for additional flavor.

Green Pepper with Sauteed Miso 257.

3 med. green peppers
1 Tbsp. sesame oil
1 heaping Tbsp. barley miso

Cut the peppers in half, remove the seeds and cut thin koguchigiri.

Heat the oil and saute the green peppers on a medium high flame in an uncovered pan until they are bright green.

Dilute the miso slightly with water and add it to the green peppers. Saute this until the miso has a fragrant smell.

Serve it either hot or cold.

Sweet Potato, Carrot and Banana Squash Nitsuke 258.

3 med. sweet potatoes, cut in half, then in 1″ strips
1 carrot, cut ¼″ sainome (diced)
2 cups banana squash, cut same as sweet potato
2 tsp. sesame oil
⅓ cup boiling water
½ tsp. sea salt

Heat the oil and saute the sweet potato for 5 minutes. Add the squash, carrot and salt. Sprinkle water around the edge of the pan. Bring to a boil covered on a high flame, then cook 20 minutes on a medium high flame.

Test the vegetables with a bamboo skewer to see if they are tender and done.

Tofu with Mustard Sauce 259.

1 block of tofu, cut in 6 pieces (see 80.)
1 Tbsp. mustard powder
1 tsp. hot green or bancha tea
1 - 4 Tbsp. tamari soy sauce

Place the 6 pieces on a plate; since tofu is quite watery, tilt the plate to one side to drain off the excess water.

Place the mustard in an oven-proof bowl and add hot tea to it. Stir quickly and invert the bowl over a burner on low heat for about 5 minutes or until the mustard mixture is slightly brown and has a strong fragrance.

Each person can mix mustard and soy sauce to his own taste. Use as a condiment with tofu. At the table, grated ginger and soy sauce is also a good condiment.

Cold, uncooked tofu tastes very good in the summer.

French-Fried Potatoes 260.

2 med. potatoes, cut into ½″ matchsticks
1 tsp. sea salt
oil for deep-frying

Mix the potatoes with the salt and let them sit for 20 minutes. Strain the excess liquid and dry the potatoes with a paper towel.

Deep-fry them until they are golden brown and serve immediately.

Note: This is the most yang style of French fries.

Goma Tofu 261.

⅓ cup sesame butter
¼ cup kuzu
½ cup boiling water
½ cup cold water

Sauce: ⅓ cup soup stock (see 80a.)
1 Tbsp. tamari soy sauce
¼ tsp. fresh ginger juice

Mix the sesame butter with the boiling water and strain it with a very fine strainer. Save what is left in the strainer for bread-making or other cooking.

Dissolve the kuzu in the cold water. Make sure you get out all the lumps. Then bring to a boil and add the sesame butter and water mixture. Boil this again and cook it 20 minutes on a medium flame, uncovered.

Pour it into a square baking dish which has been rinsed with cold water and set it aside to cool. After it has completely cooled, cut it into 1″ squares. Serve it with the sauce made from soup stock, soy sauce and ginger juice.

Fried Quail 262.

5 quail
½ cup whole wheat pastry flour
deep-frying oil

Marinade for Quail:
1 tsp. ginger juice
½ tsp. sea salt
2 tsp. tamari soy sauce
1 Tbsp. cold water or sake

Marinate the quail in the marinade sauce for 1 hour.

Then cover it with flour and let it sit for 5 minutes. Deep-fry it on a medium high flame until it is golden brown on both sides.

Parsley Miso Pickles 263a.

1 bunch parsley
2 tsp. sea salt

Wash the parsley and let it drain for ½ a day. Mix it with salt and press it in a salad press for 24 hours.

Drain and dry it completely. Place it in a cotton gauze bag, tie it and place it at the bottom of a miso keg. Cover it with miso.

When you reach the bottom of the miso, the parsley is ready — usually about 2 months.

Mince the parsley and sprinkle on curry sauce for delicious flavor.

Variation: Use shiso leaves in place of parsley. Also, shiso seeds are good in this preparation. Treat same as above.

Miso Pickles 263b.

All the following vegetables are good for this recipe: daikon, cucumber, eggplant, carrot, burdock, ginger, kombu.

Wash and clean the vegetables. Mix them with 10% of their weight in salt and put them in a container. Press them with a very heavy stone and wooden cover until the liquid comes to the top. After 24 hours, remove the vegetables.

Put 1″ of miso on the bottom of a keg. Add the vegetables in one layer and then cover them with the rest of the miso. Use the miso from this keg as usual, and when you come to a vegetable it will be ready to eat.

If you are making your own miso, put the vegetables in at the start. After 2 - 3 years you can eat them at the same time you use the miso.

Note: Use only one layer of vegetables, as too many vegetables will spoil the miso.

Kasha - Potato Croquettes

4 cups cooked kasha
2 med. potatoes
½ cup whole wheat flour
½ cup sweet brown rice flour
1 tsp. sea salt
6 Tbsp. corn oil

Pressure cook the whole potatoes for 20 minutes with 1 tsp. salt. Use a metal plate inserted into the pressure cooker on which to rest the potatoes. After they are cooked, remove the plate and mash the potatoes while they are hot.

Steam the already-cooked kasha for 20 minutes. Then add the mashed potatoes to it and set this aside to cool.

Add the whole wheat flour to the mixture and shape it into croquettes. Dust them with sweet brown rice flour and let them sit for 5 minutes. Heat 2 Tbsp. oil in a heavy skillet and place the croquettes in the skillet. Cook them 7 minutes on a medium flame in a covered pan. Then turn them over and cook until they are a golden brown.

Note: Sweet brown rice flour makes the croquettes look good. Bread crumbs, corn meal, etc., can be used instead.

Variation: Okara from making tofu can be used instead of potatoes. This is a nice combination with kasha.

Matsuba Kombu

kombu
oil for deep-frying

Choose pliable kombu and wipe it clean with a damp cloth. Cut it into 1″ × 3″ strips. Cut each strip almost in two and tie it. Move the knot up close to the end which is not cut.

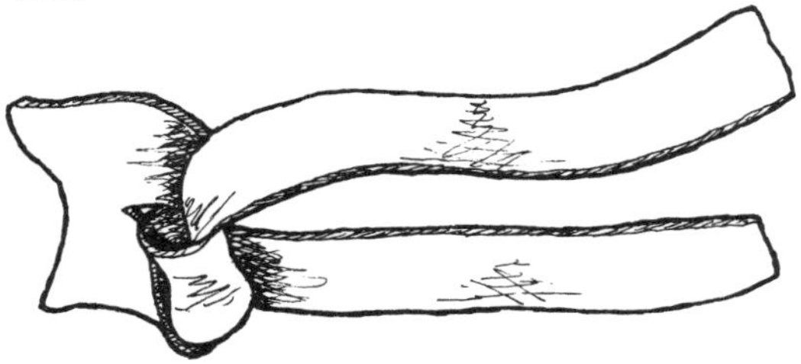

They will look like pine needles. Deep-fry them until they are crisp.

Matsuba is pine leaves. In Japan, pine, bamboo and plum blossoms are popular symbols. Pine needles come in twos, joined at the base to form a leaf. Whether on the tree or blown to the ground, you always find two together. So pine represents men and women together and is the symbol chosen for this dish.

Bamboo represents Man. It is soft and flexible yet strong and upstanding. It is evergreen. Plum blossom represents Woman. It blooms before any leaves are on the trees and while the snow is still on the ground. Though strong and hardy, like a woman it is a flower with a delicate fragrance.

Amasake Wedding Cake 266.

½ cup corn oil (not corn germ oil)
2 cups whole wheat pastry flour
1 cup amasake: warm before using and blend in blender (see 8.)
½ tsp. sea salt
½ cup warm water
1½ tsp. liquid vanilla or ½" vanilla bean
½ tsp. yeast
3 heaping Tbsp. flour

Sift the flour 3 times and add salt and oil. Use your hands to mix the oil thoroughly with the flour.

In a separate bowl add warm water to the yeast. Add to this 3 heaping Tbsp. of flour, mix well and set it aside for 15 minutes until the yeast is completely dissolved. (The flour helps to activate the yeast.) Stir this and add the warm amasake. Mix thoroughly, then add it to the flour, oil and salt mixture. Using an egg-beater or an electric beater, mix the ingredients until they form a smooth batter. Then add the vanilla. Cover the batter with a damp cloth and let it rise in a warm spot until it has doubled in size (about 1 hour).

Punch it down, place in a cake pan and cover it again. Let it rise until it doubles in size again (about 30 minutes).

Cut a brown grocery bag down the seam, open it and place the cake pan on it. Draw an outline of the bottom of the pan on the paper. Cut and place this in the bottom of the pan, which has been oiled. Pour the cake batter on top of this paper. This helps the cake bake evenly and makes it easier to remove from the pan.

Bake it at 350° about 45 - 60 minutes until it tests dry with a bamboo skewer. Remove the cake from the pan and place it on a rack to cool. Do not remove the paper until the cake has cooled. It will then peel off easily and leave an even surface.

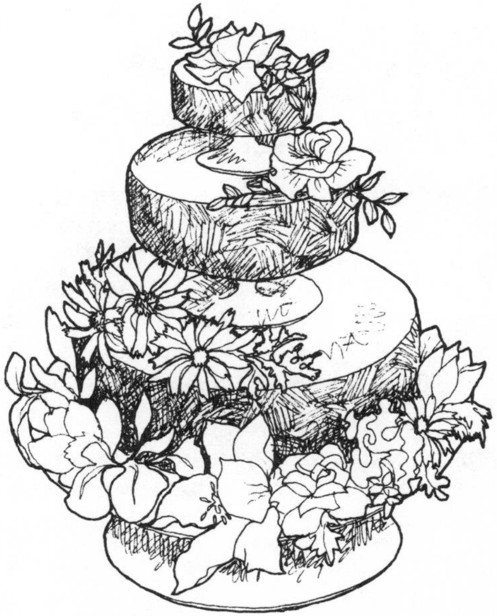

This makes an 8″ round layer cake. If you are using tiered pans, adjust the proportions according to the size of each tier. For a tiered cake, purchase heavy cardboard layer dividers from a party shop that has decorations for making home cakes for parties. To elevate between the tiers, use brandy glasses turned upside-down to support each layer, or purchase 'pillars' to use between the layers. Use bamboo skewers placed in the cake and extended into the pillars or brandy glasses to keep the cake from sliding when carrying it to the serving area.

Amasake Icing:

2 cups amasake, blended
1 tsp. kanten powder
1 tsp. grated lemon peel
½ cup water
1 tsp. vanilla
½ tsp. sea salt

Add the kanten powder to the water, bring it to a boil, then simmer it for 20 minutes in an uncovered pan with ½ tsp. salt. Skim off any foam from the top and discard it. Add the amasake and cook a few more minutes. Add the lemon peel and vanilla, mix it well, remove from heat and chill it until it sets. This does not mean that it will become firm like kanten jello; instead, it will be soft like frosting.

Before covering the cake, mix the frosting with a fork (or an egg-beater or electric mixer). Then spread it on the cake.

For special decorations, cut fruit into small pieces and use as a border design around the cake, or on top of it. If small flowers are available, use them to decorate the wedding cake.

Musubi Kombu

kombu
oil for deep-frying

Choose a pliable piece of kombu and wipe it clean with a damp cloth. Cut it into ½″×4″ strips. Tie each piece with a knot in the center (see illustration) and deep-fry them in hot oil until crisp. This happens quickly, so be careful not to burn it.

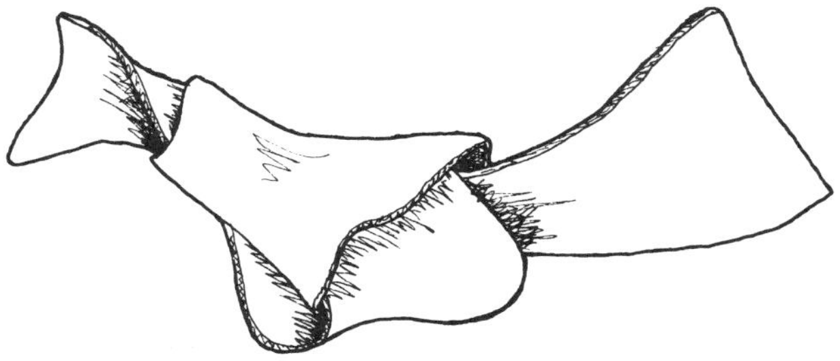

Musubi means "made by bringing yin and yang together." For example, a rice ball is *omusubi* because of the way you press your hands, one yin and one yang, together to shape the ball. In this dish it refers to the way the kombu is tied.

Kombu is used at festive occasions because 'kombu' is a similar sound to 'yorokobu,' which means 'gladness.' So you see, this is an appropriate dish to serve at a wedding.

Shad with Tomato Sauce

268.

1 shad, cut into 1″ pieces
2 cups bancha tea
3 umeboshi (salt plums)
2 pieces of sliced ginger
2 heaping Tbsp. tomato sauce (see 226.)

Place the shad in a 4-qt. pressure cooker with the umeboshi and the sliced ginger. Cover it with boiling bancha tea and pressure-cook it 3 - 4 hours.

When pressure is normal, remove the umeboshi and the ginger. Add tomato sauce to cover the fish and cook it 30 minutes without pressure.

Serve it hot or cold.

Note: To any blue-skinned fish like sardine, mackerel or shad, add a few umeboshi to take out the strong fish smell. This will give it an elegant taste.

The ginger balances the fish from a strong yang to a more pleasing and harmonious taste.

Bamboo Roll

269.

1 bunch spinach
3 sheets nori

Cook the spinach the same as ohitashi (66.).

Cut the nori in half lengthwise. Squeeze the spinach in a bamboo mat to a ½″ diameter. Place the nori on the bamboo mat and place the spinach on top. Roll this like sushi. Cut it into approximately 1″ pieces on the diagonal so that it resembles spears.

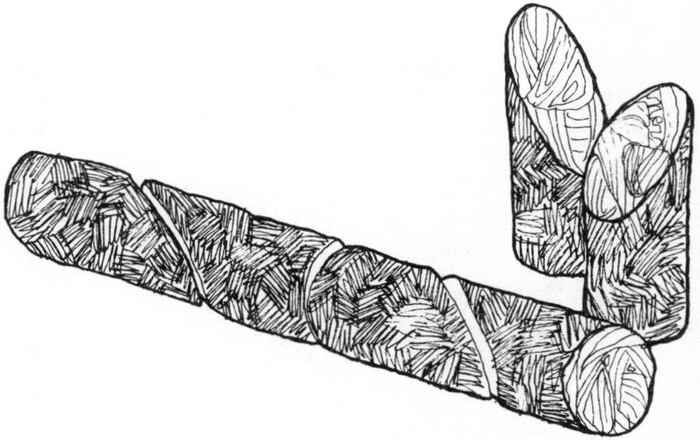

Fuku Musubi *(Tied Cabbage)* 270.

5 cabbage leaves
2″ of carrot, cut sengiri
1 onion, cut thin mawashigiri
1 slice of bread, cut ¼″ sainome
½ cup bechamel sauce (see 37a.)
1 Tbsp. chopped parsley
½ tsp. sea salt
1 cup soup stock and 1 cup water (see 16.)
1 Tbsp. tamari soy sauce
kampyo strips

Put cabbage leaves in a strainer and dip them into boiling water until they are soft.

Saute the onions, carrots and bread cubes and season them with salt. Cook these until the carrots are tender. Place a spoonful of this mixture into each cabbage leaf and fold it up into a tight package.

Rub the kampyo with warm water until it is pliable. Use this to tie up each package like a parcel. Cook the cabbage parcels in soup stock for 20 minutes, then add soy sauce to taste.

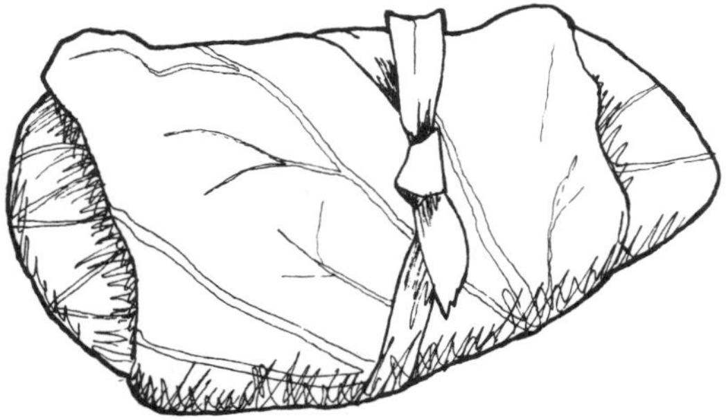

Place them on a serving dish and cover them with bechamel sauce. Garnish these with chopped parsley.

Apple Juice Drink 271.

Mix equal amounts of apple juice and bancha tea. Serve it cold.

Azuki Bean Stew 272.

1 cup azuki beans
2 onions, cut ¼″ mawashigiri
½ small cauliflower, cut into flowerettes
1 carrot, cut ichogiri
3 pieces of unyeasted bread, cut into 1″ squares
2 tsp. sea salt
1 Tbsp. tamari soy sauce
1 Tbsp. sesame oil
5 cups boiling water

Wash and soak the beans in 1⅓ cup of water overnight or at least 5 hours. Then bring them to a boil 3 times; each time add ½ cup of cold water. Cook them until they are tender — about 1 hour. Do not pressure-cook the azuki beans or they will taste bitter.

In another pot, saute the onions until they are transparent. Then add the carrots and saute them a few minutes. Add the 5 cups of boiling water and the salt and cook 10 minutes more. Add the cooked beans and bread cubes and cook 5 - 10 minutes. If necessary, add soy sauce to taste. Serve the stew hot.

Onion Soup 273.

2 med. onions, cut thin mawashigiri
1 tsp. sesame oil
¼ tsp. sea salt
5 cups boiling water
1 or 1½ Tbsp. tamari soy sauce

Saute the onions until they are transparent. Add the boiling water. Bring this to a boil with a cover and cook for 5 minutes on a medium flame. Add the salt and cook for 30 minutes on a low flame (still boiling) in a covered pot.

Add the soy sauce and bring to a boil again. Serve immediately.

Variation: Grate 1 heaping Tbsp. of cheese and add it with the soy sauce on top of the soup. Bring it to a boil and serve immediately.

Shingiku Miso Soup 274.

2″ × 2″ piece of dashi kombu
7 cups water
3 shingiku, cut into 1″ lengths
1 Tbsp. rice miso
1 Tbsp. barley miso

Soak the dashi kombu in 7 cups of water for 8 hours, or cook it for 1 hour in 7 cups of water on a low flame.

Remove the kombu and add the shingiku to the soup stock. Turn up the flame, bring it to a boil and cook for 3 minutes uncovered. Place the miso in a strainer and grind it through the strainer into the soup. Turn off the heat and serve the hot soup immediately.

Variation: Fu can be added to this soup. Cover the fu with water and soak it for 10 minutes until it is soft. Strain off the water. If it is a large piece of fu, cut it into bite-size strips after you have soaked it.

Note: If you cannot find shingiku, watercress can be substituted.

Baked Stuffed Zucchini 275.

3 med. zucchini, about 8″ long
1 cup onion-tomato sauce (see 191a.)

Cut the squash in half lengthwise and remove the seeds. Fill them with onion-tomato sauce and place on a cookie sheet or any open pan.

Bake them at 450° for 1 hour or until they are tender.

Kombu - Egg Nitsuke 276.

1 cup kombu, cut thin sengiri (can use leftover kombu from making soup stock)
1 Tbsp. tamari soy sauce
1½ cups water
1 egg, beaten

Cook the kombu with water until it is tender — about 1 hour.

Then add the soy sauce. If there is too much liquid, boil some of it away. Just a little bit should remain.

Add the egg to the kombu and mix it. When it is slightly cooked (the egg will become white), this is done.

Garlic Fried Rice 277.

3 cloves garlic, grated
3 cups bean sprouts
7 cups cooked brown rice
1 cup scallions, cut ¼″ koguchigiri
2 Tbsp. oil
1 tsp. sea salt
1 Tbsp. tamari soy sauce

Heat the oil and saute the garlic until it is slightly brown. Turn up the flame to high and saute the bean sprouts and the scallions at the same time. Then add the rice and mix it thoroughly with the vegetables. Sprinkle on the salt and when the rice is completely warmed, add the soy sauce.

Serve it immediately.

Carrot Nitsuke 278.

3 med. carrots, cut thin sengiri
2 tsp. sesame oil
1 tsp. sea salt
⅓ cup water
1 tsp. tamari soy sauce

Heat the oil and saute the carrots in a covered pan about 10 minutes, until they are slightly soft. Then add the salt and water and continue to cook them until they are tender — about 20 minutes.

Add the soy sauce to taste and serve it hot or warm.

Buckwheat Potage with Croutons 279.

1 cup buckwheat flour
7 cups water
1 tsp. sea salt
1 Tbsp. tamari soy sauce
1 tsp. sesame oil
1 Tbsp. minced parsley
Rice croutons

Heat the oil slightly and saute the buckwheat flour. Don't over-roast it, since buckwheat is very yang. Let it cool, then add the water. Be sure to mix it thoroughly. Bring this to a boil. Add the salt, cover and cook it for 20 minutes.

Add the soy sauce, bring to a boil once and serve immediately, garnished with parsley and croutons.

Rice Croutons

Take leftover rice or sour rice and wash it slightly. The rice grains will separate. Place it on a cutting board for several days to dry out completely.

Heat oil and deep-fry the rice; it will puff up. Use a strainer to scoop it out of the oil, and drain the excess oil. Be sure to fry it until it is golden brown and crisp. Sprinkle the rice on the soup with the parsley.

Variation: Add miso and sliced scallions to the potage, to taste.

Fried Chicken Wings 280.

10 chicken wings
½ cup whole wheat pastry flour
½ head lettuce, cut thin sengiri
1 orange, cut ¼″ wagiri
2 Tbsp. oil

Marinade sauce:

½ tsp. sea salt
1 tsp. ginger juice
2 tsp. tamari soy sauce
1 heaping Tbsp. minced onions

Place the chicken wings in the marinade sauce for 1 hour.

Remove them, be sure to brush off any excess onion, and dust them with flour. Let them sit for 10 minutes so that the flour is absorbed in the liquid.

Heat 2 Tbsp. oil in a pan and place the floured chicken wings in the pan. Cover and cook them for 10 minutes. Turn them over and cook for 10 minutes more, or until both sides are golden brown. Serve the chicken with chopped lettuce and the orange slices.

Fresh Corn with Onion Cream Sauce 281.

3 ears cooked corn (remove kernels with a knife)
1 med. potato, cut into bite-size pieces
5 small whole onions
1 Tbsp. minced parsley
½ cup bechamel sauce mixed with 2 cups cold water (37.)
2 tsp. sea salt
1 Tbsp. sesame oil

Saute the potato until it is slightly transparent. Add the onions, saute a few minutes, then add the corn. Cover the vegetables with boiling water and bring them to a boil. Add the salt and cook them for 30 minutes.

Then add the bechamel sauce and cook 10 minutes more. Garnish this dish with parsley.

Adjust the consistency of the sauce to your taste by increasing or decreasing the amount of water.

Konnyaku Nitsuke 282.

2 blocks konnyaku (available at Japanese stores)
1 Tbsp. sesame oil
1 Tbsp. tamari soy sauce

Cut each block of konnyaku into ½″ squares, then cut each square into very thin slices. Heat a heavy pan and add the konnyaku. Place a clean cotton kitchen towel in the pan and move it around to pick up the excess water from the konnyaku. There will be a lot of water.

When this is finished, remove the cotton cloth. Move the konnyaku to one side of the pan and add oil to the other side. Let it spread around and saute the konnyaku for 20 minutes, uncovered. Add the soy sauce and cook 20 minutes more, covered. Stir it occasionally.

Konnyaku is good for removing animal protein. It is beneficial for cleansing the intestines of deposits. It also aids the stomach and is very good for people who are too yang due to animal foods. (See *Do of Cooking - Summer,* p. 73.)

Puri 283.

3 cups whole wheat pastry flour
1 tsp. sea salt
1 cup water
oil for deep-frying

Mix the ingredients and knead them thoroughly until they have an ear lobe consistency. Roll out the dough to a ⅛″ thickness. Using a round cutter similar to a doughnut cutter, cut out round puri.

Deep-fry them in hot oil. In order to make the puri bubble, hold it under the hot oil with chopsticks after you drop it into the oil. They will puff up like a ball.

Shingiku Goma Ai *(Cooked Salad)* 284.

2 bunches shingiku
⅓ cup black or brown sesame seeds
1 tsp. barley miso
1 tsp. rice miso
2 tsp. tamari soy sauce
1 heaping tsp. sea salt
7 - 8 cups boiling water

Boil the shingiku in salted water. (Watercress can be substituted for this vegetable.) When it turns bright green and is somewhat soft, remove it and cool. Squeeze out the excess water and slice it into 1½″ strips.

Roast and grind the sesame seeds. Mix them with the miso and the soy sauce. Grind these well together, then add the shingiku to this mixture. Mix thoroughly and serve it.

Udon with Mock Meat Sauce 285.

½ lb. udon or whole wheat spaghetti
2 small onions, minced
2 Tbsp. barley miso
2 heaping Tbsp. bonita flakes
2 Tbsp. oil
5 Tbsp. water

Cook the noodles until they are tender. Strain off the water and let them drain.

Saute the onions until they are transparent, add the miso and saute them about 10 minutes more until a fragrant smell arises. Add the water and bring it to a boil. Add the bonita flakes and the cooked noodles. Mix thoroughly and serve immediately.

This dish appeals to those who are beginning macrobiotics. It helps them become more familiar with miso and its uses.

Shingiku - Endive Norimaki 286.

1 bunch endive
1 bunch shingiku (or any green vegetable)
3 sheets nori
1 Tbsp. brown or white sesame seeds, roasted
salted water

Boil the endive and the shingiku separately in salted water, in uncovered pots, so that their color becomes bright green. Let them cool. (See 66.)

Then roll each separately in a sushi mat and squeeze out the excess water. Place a sheet of nori on top of a bamboo mat, with a layer of shingiku and a layer of endive on top. Roll it similar to making norimaki sushi (see 146.).

Chop up the roasted sesame seeds into smaller pieces with a knife.

Slice each roll in 1″ wagiri and sprinkle the cut side with sesame seeds. Serve them cool.

Pan-Fried Mochi with Nori 287.

10 pieces of cold mochi (see 2A)
2 Tbsp. oil
3 sheets nori, cut into 12 pieces
2 Tbsp. tamari soy sauce

Heat a frying pan. Add the oil and the cold mochi. Cover and cook them over a medium flame for 7 minutes. The mochi should puff slightly. Turn them over and cook a few minutes more.

Place soy sauce in a dish, turn the mochi in the soy sauce and then cover it with nori.

Serve it hot.

Buckwheat Macaroni Soup 288.

2 med. onions, cut thin mawashigiri
¼ head cabbage, cut thin sengiri
1 stalk celery, cut thin hasugiri
2″ of carrot, cut thin sengiri
1 Tbsp. sesame oil
1 tsp. sea salt
2 Tbsp. tamari soy sauce
2 cups buckwheat macaroni
8 cups boiling water
1 heaping Tbsp. chopped scallions

Saute the onions, cabbage, celery and carrot separately in that order. Add the boiling water and bring it to a boil. Add the salt and washed macaroni and cook until the macaroni is tender.

Add the soy sauce to season, bring the soup to a boil, and serve it hot. Garnish this with chopped scallions.

Burdock, Carrot, Fresh Mushroom Nitsuke 289.

2 med. burdock, cut sasagaki
3 carrots, cut sasagaki
1 cup fresh mushrooms
1 Tbsp. sesame oil
½ tsp. sea salt
1 Tbsp. tamari soy sauce

Soak the mushrooms in salted water for 20 minutes. Wash, then slice them into bite-size pieces.

Saute the burdock in a covered pan about 5 minutes. Dip a wooden spoon into the salt, then stir the burdock. Cover it again and cook for 5 minutes. Repeat this salting procedure 2 more times. After 15 minutes the burdock will have a sweet smell.

Add the mushrooms and saute them for a few minutes. Then add the carrots and saute them a few minutes. Add the salt and soy sauce. Cover and cook the nitsuke on a low flame for 10 minutes. Water will be drawn from the vegetables. Cook this on a medium flame until the vegetables are tender.

Tofu with Kuzu Sauce 290.

½ block tofu, cut into 1″ pieces
2 med. zucchini, cut ½″ wagiri
2 onions, cut thin mawashigiri
1 heaping Tbsp. arrowroot flour
5 cups boiling water
½ tsp. sea salt
1 Tbsp. sesame oil
2 Tbsp. tamari soy sauce

Saute the onions until they are transparent. Add the zucchini and cook it until its color changes. Add the salt and boiling water and cook these for 20 minutes with the pan covered.

Dissolve the arrowroot in cold water and add it to the vegetables. The liquid will become thicker.

Add the tofu and the soy sauce, bring everything to a boil and serve the dish immediately.

Udon Sukiyaki with Mock Chicken 291.

5 small whole onions
2 zucchini, cut ½″ wagiri
1 block tofu, cut into 1″ squares
5 pieces of mock chicken
5 Chinese cabbage rolls (see 123.)
5 whole mushrooms (cook 10 min. in 1 cup water and 1 tsp. tamari)
½ lb. udon (white noodles)
8 cups soup stock (see 16.)
1 tsp. sea salt
¼ cup tamari soy sauce

Mock Chicken: 1 cup burdock, cut mijingiri
1 cup onion, cut mijingiri
1 cup whole wheat pastry flour
1 cup water
1 tsp. sea salt
oil for deep-frying

For mock chicken: Mix the flour, water and 1 tsp. salt, like a tempura batter; then add the vegetables. Heat the oil and deep-fry the mixture, dropping it by the spoonful into the hot oil. Cook until it is crisp.

Heat the soup stock in a shallow pan. Add 1 tsp. salt and the soy sauce. Cook the onions and the zucchini in the stock until they are tender.

Prepare the udon. Place the cooked noodles on one side of the pan and bring to a boil. Add the tofu, mock chicken, cabbage rolls and mushrooms in that order and bring this to a boil (to warm the vegetables). Turn flame off.

Serve this immediately, placing noodles, cabbage rolls, vegetables, tofu and mock chicken for each person in a shallow bowl with some soup stock. Keep each item separate.

Whole Wheat Bread 292.

6 cups whole wheat flour
2 cups unbleached white flour
½ tsp. yeast
2½ cups warm water
1 Tbsp. sea salt
1 Tbsp. oil

In ½ cup of warm water, dissolve the yeast completely. Leave this in a warm place for 5 minutes and add 2 heaping Tbsp. of flour. It will be like a tempura batter. Let it sit in a warm spot until it bubbles.

In 2 cups of warm water, mix the oil and salt. Add the yeast mixture to the flours, then add the salt and oil mixture. Knead the dough until it has an ear lobe consistency. Then cover the bowl with a wet towel and let sit in a warm place 4 hours (or until the bread dough doubles in size).

Punch it down and let it rise again (about 1 hour).

Make 2 loaves, put them in a cold oven and bake them at 450° for 45 minutes to 1 hour.

Apricot Kanten 293.

1 cup dried apricots
1 heaping Tbsp. kanten powder or 2 bars kanten
5 cups cold water
1 tsp. sea salt
7 yinnies

Soak the apricots in 2 cups of water until they are soft — about 1 hour. Then cook them for 20 minutes.

Mix 3 cups of cold water with the kanten powder and salt. Bring it to a boil in an uncovered pan and add 7 yinnie pieces in the water. Cook this 20 minutes. If a foam appears on top, skim it off.

Add the cooked apricots and cook the kanten 5 more minutes. Then pour it into a mold, chill it until it hardens, and cut and serve.

Soybean Nitsuke 294.

½ cup soybeans, dry roasted (no oil) until brown
1 med. burdock, cut rangiri
1 med. carrot, cut rangiri
3″ × 6″ piece of dashi kombu, cut into 1″ squares
2 tsp. sesame oil
1 Tbsp. tamari soy sauce

Soak the kombu in 2 cups of water. Heat the oil in a pressure cooker and saute the burdock about 7 minutes. Add the soybeans, saute them a few minutes, then add the kombu and water. Pressure-cook this for 20 minutes.

Let the pressure come down, remove cover and add the carrot. Cover the cooker and bring it to pressure again. When the gauge jiggles, shut off flame and let the pressure return to normal. Add the soy sauce and cook the nitsuke 20 minutes without pressure.

Baked Fresh Tuna 295.

5 pieces fresh tuna
1 Tbsp. ginger juice
2 tsp. sea salt
1″ of daikon, grated

Place the fish on a plate, squeeze ginger juice over it and sprinkle on 1 tsp. of salt. Let sit for 20 minutes.

Oil a cookie sheet, preheat it 5 minutes in a 450° oven and place the tuna on it. About 10″ above the fish, sprinkle on 1 tsp. salt with your fingers. After it is baked, the salt will give a nice white color.

Bake it about 20 - 30 minutes and serve it with grated daikon.

Apple Butter Kanten 296.

1 heaping Tbsp. kanten powder or 2 bars kanten
4 cups water
1½ cups apple butter (see 152.)
1 tsp. sea salt
2 cups sliced, peeled, bite-size apples

Mix the water and kanten powder, bring it to a boil and add the salt and apples. Lower the flame and cook for 15 minutes.

Add the apple butter and cook it 5 minutes more, stirring frequently. Place it in a mold and let it chill. Serve when it is firm.

Chick Pea with Sweet Rice 297.

2 cups brown rice
1 cup sweet brown rice
4 cups water
½ cup chick peas
½ tsp. sea salt

Mix the rice and chick peas together. Wash them and let them soak in 4 cups of water for 8 hours. Cook them as in 1a.

Variation: Pinto beans, green peas, white beans or kidney beans can be used. Prepare them the same as the chick peas.

Dandelion Root - Burdock Nitsuke 298.

1 cup burdock, cut sasagaki
1/3 cup dandelion root, cut thin koguchigiri
1 Tbsp. sesame oil
1 Tbsp. tamari soy sauce
2 Tbsp. boiling water

Heat the oil and saute the dandelion root in a covered pan. Cook it for 5 minutes on a low flame, then turn it over and cook it for 5 minutes again. Add the burdock and keep it covered. Cook 5 minutes, turn it over and cook another 5 minutes.

Add the soy sauce and water and cook it on a low flame until the vegetables are tender (about 30 minutes). Add more liquid if necessary.

Scallion Condiment 299.

½ cup thinly sliced scallions
2 sheets roasted nori, crushed
1 heaping Tbsp. bonita flakes
1 Tbsp. tamari soy sauce

Mix all of the above and serve it as a condiment for rice. This is a good appetizer for food.

Mustard Green and Onion Nitsuke 300.

1 bunch mustard greens, stems cut 1″ koguchigiri, leaves cut 1½″ koguchigiri, then cut across
3 med. onions, cut ¼″ mawashigiri
1 Tbsp. sesame oil
¼ tsp. sea salt
1 Tbsp. tamari soy sauce

Remove the spoiling leaves from the mustard before washing it. Fill a large container with cold water and wash the mustard greens, especially the inside of the stems. Wash them quickly and let them drain.

Heat the oil and saute the onions until they are transparent. Add the stems and cook them uncovered until they turn bright green. Add the leaves and cook them until they too become bright green. Add the salt and the soy sauce. Stir and continue to cook the vegetables until they are tender.

Sauteed Apples and Pumpkin 301.

3 cups sliced, peeled, bite-size apples
1½ cups sliced pumpkin (remove outer skin and cut into bite-size pieces)
½ tsp. sea salt
2 tsp. oil
1 tsp. cinnamon

Saute the apples until they are transparent. Add the pumpkin and saute it covered. Water will come from them. Add the salt and continue to saute, covered. Stir occasionally.

After 20 minutes, test the pumpkin for tenderness. Add the cinnamon and cook it a few minutes more. Chill and serve it cool.

The pumpkin will have a taste similar to pineapple.

Parsnip, Beet Nitsuke 302.

3 parsnips, cut in half-moon ½″
1 beet, cut in half-moon ¼″
1 tsp. sesame oil
½ tsp. sea salt
⅓ cup boiling water

Saute the parsnips in an uncovered pressure cooker. After a few minutes, add the beets and saute a few more minutes. Add the boiling water and salt, cover and cook under pressure for 5 minutes.

Let the pressure return to normal and serve it hot.

Stuffed Acorn Squash 303.

3 med. acorn squash
3 med. onions, cut thin mawashigiri
3 med. carrots, cut thin hasugiri
½ small cabbage, cut thin sengiri
⅓ cup home-made seitan, cut into small pieces (see 87a.)
2 tsp. sea salt
2 Tbsp. sesame oil
1 cup unbleached white flour
1 egg
1½ cups cold water

Cut the squash in half, remove the seeds and make a flat spot on the outer skin so that it does not wobble.

Heat 1 Tbsp. of oil. Roast the flour until it is fragrant, then allow to cool. Mix it with cold water when it has cooled.

Heat the remaining Tbsp. oil and saute the onions, cabbage and carrot. Then add the salt and the seitan. Cook this 10 minutes, then cool.

Beat the egg and combine it with the cooled, roasted flour. Mix this with the sauteed vegetables and seitan. Stuff this into the squash and brush the edge of the squash with oil.

Preheat the oven to 450° and bake the squash 1 hour.

Kombu, Dried Tofu, Age Nitsuke 304.

4 oz. kombu, cut into pieces 1″ square
3 pieces dried tofu, cut into ¼″ tanzaku
5 pieces home-made age, cut sengiri (see 64.)
1 Tbsp. tamari soy sauce

Cover the kombu with water and soak it 10 minutes. Strain the water through a cotton cloth and save it.

Place the dried tofu in hot water. After 10 minutes, squeeze the water from the tofu — it will have a white color. Repeat this process by changing the water and squeezing the tofu until the water is clear. It will take about 5 - 6 times. Cut the tofu.

Place the kombu, dried tofu and reserved kombu-soaking water in a pressure cooker and pressure-cook them 15 minutes.

When the pressure returns to normal, remove the cover and add the age. Bring this to a boil, add soy sauce and cook 20 minutes more without pressure.

Millet and Soybean Soup 305a.

1 cup millet
¼ cup soybeans
2 med. onions, cut thin mawashigiri
1 turnip, cut into bite-size pieces
½ stalk celery, cut hasugiri
2 tsp. sea salt
1 Tbsp. sesame oil
1 Tbsp. tamari soy sauce
2 cups boiling water
6 cups boiling water

Wash the soybeans and soak them in ½ cup of water for 5 hours. Grind them in a blender or suribachi.

Wash the millet and cook it in 2 cups of boiling water under pressure for 20 minutes.

Heat the oil and saute the onions, turnip, celery and carrot. Add 6 cups of boiling water, bring to a boil and cook for 20 minutes. Add salt and the cooked millet and cook this for 20 minutes. Add the blended soybeans and cook 10 minutes. Then add soy sauce to taste.

Serve this soup hot.

Millet Soup 305b.

1 cup millet
1 med. onion, cut mawashigiri
½ small cabbage, cut into 1″ squares
1 stalk celery, cut hasugiri
½ carrot, cut ichogiri
1 Tbsp. sesame oil
7 cups boiling water
2 cups boiling water
2 tsp. sea salt
1 tsp. tamari soy sauce

Wash the millet and cook it in 2 cups of boiling water in a pressure cooker for 20 minutes.

Heat the oil in another pan and saute the onion, cabbage, celery and carrot. Add 7 cups of boiling water and cook for 20 minutes. Add the salt and the millet and cook 20 minutes more.

Add the soy sauce and serve the soup hot.

Vegetable Raisin Pie 306.

2 cups leftover sauteed apples and pumpkin (see 301.)
1 cup leftover parsnip and beet nitsuke (see 302.)
2 Tbsp. raisins
pie shell (see 31.)

Mix all of the above filling ingredients.

Make a pie shell including cinnamon in your ingredients.

Put the mixture into the pie shell and bake the pie at 450° for 45 minutes.

Wild Scallion and Seitan Nitsuke 307.

2 cups wild scallions, cut in 1″ strips
1/3 cup seitan, cut thin (see 87.)
1 Tbsp. sesame oil
1 tsp. tamari soy sauce

Heat the oil and saute the wild scallions using a high flame. When the color of the vegetables changes to bright green, add the seitan and the soy sauce. Cover and cook the nitsuke for 10 minutes.

Serve it hot.

Vegetable Pie 308.

6 med. onions, cut thin mawashigiri
1 med. carrot, cut thin hasugiri
1 bunch scallions, cut 1/4″ koguchigiri
2 eggs, beaten
3/4 cup water
1/4 cup unbleached white flour
1 1/2 tsp. sea salt
2 tsp. oil

Pie Crust: 3 cups whole wheat pastry flour
3 Tbsp. oil
1/2 tsp. sea salt
1 cup cold water

Heat the oil and saute the onions and carrot. Add the salt and water and cook the vegetables for 15 minutes. Sprinkle on the scallions, take the pot off the flame and let it cool.

When the vegetables are completely cooled, add the beaten egg. Sprinkle the flour in this mixture and be careful not to get it lumpy.

Make the pie shell, put the mixture in the shell and bake 45 minutes at 450°.

Steamed Cabbage 309.

1 med. cabbage, cut into 1″ squares
1/2 to 1 tsp. sea salt
1/4 cup boiling water

Use a heavy pan. Put the cabbage leaves in the pan and add 1 cup of boiling water around the edge of the pan. Sprinkle salt on top of the cabbage. Cook the cabbage on a medium flame for 20 minutes, covered.

Turn it over and cook it 10 minutes more on a medium flame. If necessary, add more water.

Cranberry Sauce 310a.

3 lbs. cranberries
4 apples, cut thinly
1 lb. raisins
7 cups apple cider

Cook all of the above for 1 hour in an uncovered pot, then blend them together in a blender.

Cook them again until the sauce is thick and creamy. Serve cold.

Raw Cranberry Sauce 310b.

4 cups cranberries
2 large oranges
½ cup apple cider

Slice the oranges into quarters, remove all seeds and blend them together with the other ingredients. Let this sit overnight and serve it cool.

Cranberry Sauce Variation 310c.

7 cups cranberries
4 cups apples, thinly sliced
1 tsp. sesame oil
1½ cups water

Saute the apples about 7 minutes, then add the water and washed cranberries. Cook this in an uncovered pan for 2 hours, then blend in a food mill.

Cool this by letting it sit overnight.

Lotus Root Nitsuke 311.

1 cup lotus root, cut thin wagiri
1 tsp. sesame oil
¼ tsp. sea salt
1 Tbsp. tamari soy sauce
½ cup boiling water

Heat the oil and saute the lotus root for 5 minutes. Add salt and water and cook it covered for 30 minutes.

Add soy sauce and cook 20 minutes more. Add more water if necessary.

Do not cook the lotus root until it is too soft — it is better if it is a little crisp.

Whole Wheat Buns 312.

12 cups whole wheat flour
3 cups unbleached white flour
3 cups brown rice flour
2½ Tbsp. oil
2 Tbsp. sea salt
6 cups warm water

Yeast mixture:

½ cup warm water
1 tsp. yeast
2 heaping Tbsp. white flour

Dissolve the yeast in the ½ cup of warm water and mix in 2 heaping Tbsp. white flour. Let sit in warm place for 10 minutes until the mixture bubbles.

Mix the water, oil and salt with an egg beater. Mix this with the flours and add the yeast mixture to this. (Use some of the oil-water mixture to get all of the yeast from the bowl.)

Stir the batter with a wooden spoon until all the ingredients are mixed thoroughly. Cover the bowl with a wet cloth and place in a warm spot. Let the dough double in size (about 4 hours).

Wet your hands and punch down the dough. Turn the top of the dough to the bottom and let it rise a second time (about 1 hour).

Sprinkle corn meal in a 2″-high cake pan or sheet. Wet your hands and make buns 1″ in diameter. Place them close together on the cake sheet in a cold oven. Turn the oven to 450° and bake them for 1 hour or until the tops are slightly brown.

Variation: Sprinkle the tops with poppy seeds or sesame seeds.

Brussels Sprouts - Beet Salad with Mayonnaise 313.

3 lbs. Brussels sprouts
3 med. beets, whole
8 cups boiling water
1 heaping tsp. sea salt

Remove the outer leaves of the Brussels sprouts and cook sprouts in salted water for about 10 minutes in an uncovered pan on a high flame. They should be tender but still crisp. Drain the excess water and let them cool.

Place the beets on a vegetable steamer in a pressure cooker and pressure-cook for 20 minutes. Let the pressure come down and cool the beets. Cut them into ¼″ slices (wagiri) and serve beets and sprouts with mayonnaise dressing.

Dressing: 3 eggs
1½ cups cool, cooked oil
4 tsp. sea salt
1 Tbsp. lemon juice, if necessary
1 cup tangerine juice, if necessary

Put the eggs and 2 tsp. of salt into a blender and blend the following: Add ½ cup of oil by letting it drip off a chopstick, then add the remaining salt. Add ½ cup of oil by teaspoon; add the last ½ cup by tablespoon. If it is too thick, add lemon juice to thin it. If it continues to be thick, add the tangerine juice.

If you desire, add white pepper to taste.

If you have no blender, use an egg beater. Be sure that the egg beater, bowl and ingredients stay cool before making mayonnaise.

Pumpkin Pie 314.

Filling: 2 tsp. sea salt
3½ lbs. Hokkaido pumpkin or any sweet winter squash
2 tsp. cinnamon
1 tsp. nutmeg
½ tsp. vanilla
2 eggs
a little oil

Cut the skin from the pumpkin or squash and scrape out all the seeds and lining. Cut it into ½″ pieces and saute them in a little oil for about 15 minutes. Add 1 cup of water and pressure-cook them for 30 minutes with 2 tsp. of salt. Reduce the pressure and remove the pumpkin from the pot. Cool it 30 minutes. Then put it through a food mill. During this blending process, add the beaten eggs, cinnamon, nutmeg and vanilla.

Pie Crust: 1½ cups whole wheat pastry flour
1½ cups bran flour
3 cups unbleached white flour
½ tsp. sea salt
1¼ cups corn oil
¾ cup water

Combine the flours in a mixing bowl and add the salt. Add the oil, rubbing it by hand until it is completely mixed with the flour. Mix in the water with a fork — do not knead. Roll the dough thinly and place it into pie pans. Bake in a 350° oven for 10 minutes — until pie shells are slightly brown. Remove from the oven and let cool before adding the filling. (This makes 4 pie shells, so you may have an extra shell to use for your favorite recipe.)

Fill the pie shells generously with the cooled pumpkin mixture. Bake the pies in a 350 - 375° oven for about 30 minutes, until each is golden brown. Cool them before serving.

This tastes like old-fashioned pumpkin pie. It is delicious.

Tangerine Kanten

1½ cups tangerine juice
2 kanten bars
2 cups water
⅓ cup yinnie syrup or honey
1 tsp. sea salt

Wash the kanten in cold water and soak for 5 minutes. Bring the water and kanten to a boil and add the salt. Cook it for 15 minutes in an uncovered pot.

When white foam comes to the surface, skim it off.

Add the yinnie syrup (or honey), cook 5 more minutes and then turn it off. When the mixture is body temperature, mix in the tangerine juice.

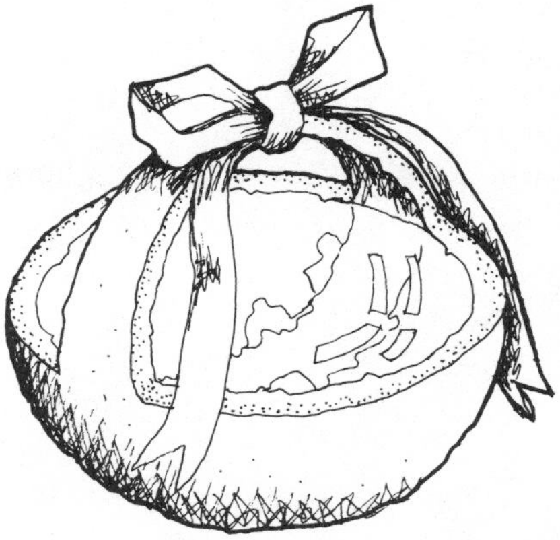

To serve: Cut the tangerines so that they look like little baskets. Remove the inner pulp to use for juice. Pour some of the kanten into the tangerine baskets and let it become firm. These can be used as decorations and are nice for children's birthday parties.

Country Potage 316.

2 onions, cut thin mawashigiri
½ carrot, cut ichogiri
½ stalk celery, cut thinly
2 turnips, cut in bite-size pieces
2 stalks broccoli
¼ cup rice cream, uncooked
1 Tbsp. sesame oil
2 tsp. sea salt
1 tsp. tamari soy sauce
4 cups boiling water

Boil the broccoli in salted water until it is tender on a high flame in an uncovered pot. Remove and let it cool. Separate flowerettes from stem. (Use the water for soup.)

Saute the onions, turnip, celery and carrot for a few minutes. Add the boiling water and cook the vegetables until they are tender. Blend all of them finely, and mix in the rice cream. Bring this to a boil and cook 20 minutes.

Season it with soy sauce and serve, adding pieces of broccoli in each bowl.

Watercress Nitsuke 317.

2 bunches watercress, cut in 1″ strips
1 tsp. sesame oil
2 tsp. tamari soy sauce

Heat the oil and saute the watercress on a high flame until it turns bright green. Add the soy sauce, cook it a few minutes and serve it hot or cool.

Watercress is a very yang vegetable; don't overcook it. Be sure to not use a cover when cooking or it will lose its bright green color.

Stuffed Green Peppers 318.

5 med. green peppers
2 cups turkey stuffing (166.) or cooked kasha (24.)
2″ × 3″ dashi kombu
2 cups boiling water
1 tsp. sea salt
½ cup roasted and cooled whole wheat pastry flour
2 tsp. tamari soy sauce

Cut the tops off the green peppers (about ¼″) and reserve them for covers. Remove the seeds from inside the peppers. Stuff the peppers with kasha or turkey stuffing.

Place the kombu on the bottom of a pan and place the stuffed peppers in the pan, using their reserved tops as covers. Add the salt to the boiling water and add to the pan. Cook 20 minutes over a medium flame.

Mix the roasted flour with ½ cup of cold water. Remove the peppers from the pan. Add the flour mixture to the pan and mix. Bring this to a boil and cook for 10 minutes. Add soy sauce to taste, then pour this sauce over the stuffed green peppers and serve them hot.

Currant Kanten 319.

3 cups water
2 cups fresh tangerine juice
5 cups water
2 heaping Tbsp. kanten powder or 4 kanten bars
2 cups currants
2 tsp. sea salt
prune and cherry pits

Mix 3 cups of water with prune and cherry pits left over from making fruit cake (334.). Soak them 1 hour, then strain off the liquid and reserve.

Dissolve the kanten powder in 5 cups of water and add the currants, salt and the fruit water. Cook this for 20 minutes. Let it cool until body temperature. Add the tangerine juice and mix well.

Place it in a mold and let it cool. Serve it chilled.

Cucumber Mustard Pickles 320.

36 pickling cucumbers
1 cup sea salt
3 Tbsp. mustard powder
3 cups amasake (see 8.)
1½ Tbsp. green or bancha tea

After washing the cucumbers, dry them and put them in a vegetable press for 24 hours with salt (see 263b.).

Make about 1 cup of strong tea. Place the mustard powder in an oven-proof bowl. Add 1½ Tbsp. of hot tea and stir it quickly. Then, invert the bowl over a burner on low heat for about 5 minutes, or until mustard mixture is slightly browned and there is a potent mustard aroma. Add the amasake to the mustard.

On the bottom of a clean porcelain or glass container, place about 3 Tbsp. of the mustard mixture and add a layer of cucumber. Alternate layers of cucumber and mustard until all the cucumbers are used. Cover the container and keep it in the refrigerator 1 to 1½ months.

These pickles will then be ready to eat. They are delicious with fried foods.

Variation: After the mustard and tea mixture has been 'fired,' add a little bit of soy sauce to it. This is good on cooked vegetables and pressed green salad.

Note: Do not eat mustard if you are troubled with hemorrhoids.

Cracked Wheat with Onions 321.

2 cups cracked wheat
2 onions, cut thin mawashigiri
½ tsp. sea salt
2 tsp. oil
6 cups boiling water

Heat 1 tsp. of oil and saute the cracked wheat until it is slightly colored and fragrant.

Saute the onions in a separate pan with 1 tsp. of oil. When the onions are transparent, add the salt and the boiling water. Cover this and bring to a boil. Add the cracked wheat and cook on a low flame, stirring occasionally. Add more water if necessary.

(A pinch of thyme, basil or garlic can be added to enhance the flavor.)

Baked Rice with Walnut and Seitan 322.

3 cups roasted brown rice
$2/3$ cup seitan, cut thinly (see 87a.)
$2/3$ cup chopped walnuts
1 - 4 tsp. tamari soy sauce
6 cups boiling water

Mix all of the above ingredients and bake them at 350° for one hour.

Mix thoroughly and serve it hot. Use chopped parsley for a garnish.

Rice Patties 323.

2 cups cooked rice
½ cup water
1 heaping Tbsp. barley miso
½ cup whole wheat pastry flour
2 Tbsp. corn oil
1 small onion, cut mijingiri

Dissolve the miso in water and add the rice. Break it into smaller pieces with a rice paddle, then add the flour. Mix these well. Add more flour if the mixture is too moist.

Spoon the mixture into flat patties. Cook them in a hot oiled heavy frying pan with a cover for 7 minutes (on medium heat) on each side, until both sides are a golden brown color.

Serve them immediately.

Turnip, Turnip Top and Sake-Kasu Nitsuke 324.

3 med. turnips, cut ¼″ mawashigiri
3 turnip tops, cut in 1″ strips
1 heaping Tbsp. chirimen iriko (small dried fish)
1 Tbsp. sesame oil
½ cup sake-kasu (available from Japanese food stores)
½ cup boiling water
½ tsp. sea salt
1 Tbsp. tamari soy sauce

Dilute the sake-kasu with the boiling water.

Saute the turnip tops until they are bright green. Add the turnips, chirimen iriko, salt and soy sauce and cook on a medium flame for 15 minutes (until the vegetables are half done). Add the sake-kasu and cook it 20 minutes more.

This dish is good on cold days. It keeps the body warm for a long time.

Fried Oysters with Fried Saifun 325.

15 medium-size oysters
4 oz. saifun (see 88.)
1 head lettuce, cut ¼" sengiri
1 lemon, cut into 6 half-moon slices
2 eggs, beaten
2 cups bread crumbs
⅓ cup whole wheat pastry flour
1 Tbsp. sea salt
oil for deep-frying

Place some cold water with salt in a pot large enough for a strainer. Place the oysters in the strainer and swish the strainer in the water. After washing the oysters, let the water drain off.

Dust them in flour, dip them in the egg and cover them with bread crumbs. Flatten the oysters slightly with your hand as you cover them with the bread crumbs. Let them sit for 10 minutes, so that the bread crumbs will absorb the liquid.

Heat the oil for deep-frying. Pick up 10 strings of dry saifun and place them in the hot oil. Stir with chopsticks to shape them into a spiral (see 88.). Make 5 rolls and set them aside to drain off the excess oil.

Place the oysters in the hot oil and cook them until they are slightly crisp on both sides. Don't overcook the oysters or they will shrink.

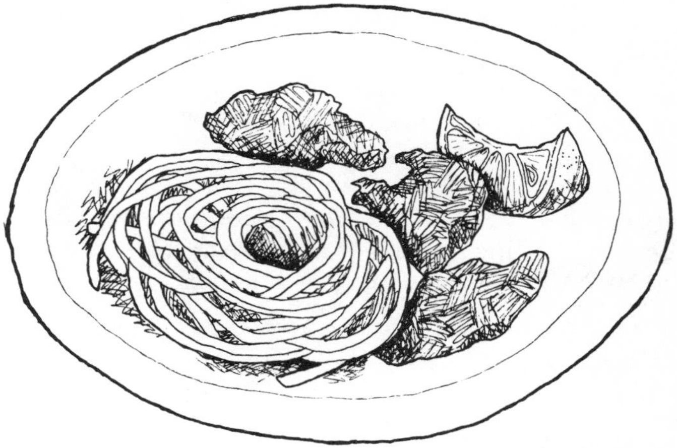

When serving them, place 3 oysters, a piece of lettuce and then a spiral of saifun on each plate. Add a slice of lemon on the side.

Oysters are good for people with lung problems and this is a nice dish to serve in the winter. It creates energy. Oysters have a lot of iron, which helps to manufacture hemoglobin.

Oysters are the most yin shellfish; they never move, thus they are similar to a vegetable.

If your body is weak and the temperature is cold, this dish will make you feel more energetic. It is most satisfying and attractive to serve, especially on a cold day.

Mixed Dried Fruit Kanten 326.

1½ cups apricots
½ cup prunes
5 dates, chopped
5 cups water
1 heaping Tbsp. kanten powder or 2 kanten bars
1 tsp. sea salt

Dissolve the kanten in cold water and add all the ingredients. Bring this to a boil in an uncovered pot and cook it on a low flame for 20 minutes.

Place it in a mold to cool and set, then serve it.

Kombu Roll 327.

3″ × 12″ piece of nishime kombu
1 carrot, quartered lengthwise
1 burdock, quartered lengthwise
2 Tbsp. tamari soy sauce
3 cups water from soaking kombu
8 strips of kampyo, 6″ long

Soak the kombu in water until it is easy to handle. Soak the kampyo in water in another bowl.

Place a strip of kombu on a flat surface and arrange the vegetable strips along its length. Roll it tightly twice and tie it in two evenly-spaced places with the kampyo strips. Repeat this for the other rolls.

Place the rolls in a pressure cooker and add soaking water to cover them. Pressure-cook them for 30 minutes. After the pressure returns to normal, add soy sauce and cook them on a low flame for 10 minutes.

(If you do not use a pressure cooker, cook in a sauce pan for 1 hour, then add soy sauce and cook another half hour.)

Cut each roll in 2 serving pieces.

Parsnip - Watercress Nitsuke 328.

1 bunch watercress, cut in 1″ lengths
3 med. parsnips, cut 1½″ wagiri, then into half-moons
½ tsp. sea salt
1 tsp. tamari soy sauce

Place the parsnips in a pressure cooker. Cover them with ¼ cup of boiling water and sprinkle on ½ tsp. salt. Cook them under pressure for 5 minutes. When the pressure returns to normal, remove the cover and sprinkle on the soy sauce. Add the watercress and cook these for a few minutes only, until the watercress becomes bright green.

Watercress complements the flavor of parsnips. This is a good combination.

Amasake Crescent Cookies 329.

4 cups whole wheat pastry flour
4 Tbsp. oil
1 tsp. sea salt
1 cup + 2 Tbsp. water
1 cup amasake concentrate (see 8.)
½ tsp. grated lemon rind

Mix the amasake concentrate and the lemon rind together.

Mix the flour, oil and salt with your hands. Add the water and mix this with a fork. Roll this dough out thin and cut it into strips 5″ wide. From these strips, cut triangles with a 4″ base. Place ½ tsp. of amasake concentrate at the base of each triangle. Roll them up and shape them into crescents, using water if necessary to seal the top of the triangles.

Dust a cookie sheet with corn meal and bake the cookies for 30 minutes at 450°.

Variation: 4 cups unbleached white flour
1 tsp. lemon rind
4 Tbsp. oil
1 cup + 4 Tbsp. water

These can be substituted in the above recipe.

Amasake concentrate: After blending amasake, cook it uncovered. Slowly the amasake will become brown until it has a consistency like apple butter. You can keep this concentrate stored for 1 month. It is good for babies who are being weaned, and can be put in kokkoh or made into a kuzu sauce to be used as a general sweetener.

Takana Pressed Salad 330.

1 bunch takana (Japanese mustard green)
2 tsp. sea salt

Wash the takana, then let it drain for half a day.

Cut it into 1″ lengths and mix it with the salt. Put it in a salad press and apply pressure to it. Let it sit in a cool place until the water comes out of the vegetable.

You can eat it about 5 hours later but it is more tasty after 2 days.

Toasted Nori 331.

Take 2 sheets of nori sea weed and put them together with their shiny sides touching. Over a medium flame, gently but quickly move the nori. Continue this until the nori changes its color to slightly green.

Roast only the outer sides of the nori.

Cut the nori in half lengthwise, then cut the halves again lengthwise. After this, cut the lengths into 2″ squares.

Serve the nori with tamari soy sauce.

Pan-Fried Cod 332.

2 lbs. cod fish (or any fillet)
⅓ cup whole wheat pastry flour
2 Tbsp. oil

Marinade: 2 tsp. ginger juice
3 Tbsp. tamari soy sauce
3 Tbsp. sake

Slice fillet, which is about 1″ thick, into 3″ pieces; cut on the diagonal (hasugiri). Marinate the fish for 15 minutes. Remove it from the marinade and dust it with flour. Let fish sit for 5 minutes.

Heat the oil in a frying pan, add the fish and cook it covered until one side is brown. Turn the fish over and cook it uncovered until the other side is brown also.

To serve it, place the cooked fish onto sliced lettuce and decorate the edge of the plate with red radishes cut into flower shapes.

To make the radish flowers, place the radish on the cutting board and keep the tip of your knife on the board. Don't let the tip move, as you cut the radish almost all the way through. Cut lines across it ⅛″ apart. Turn the radish and cut lines again so that it looks like a grille. Place into ice water and the radishes will open like a flower.

Tofu - Egg Clear Soup with Watercress *(serves 20)* 333.

10 cups soup stock (80a.)
10 cups water
1 block tofu, cut ¼″ sainome (see 80.)
1 bunch watercress, cut in 1″ lengths
1 egg, beaten
3 Tbsp. tamari soy sauce
4 tsp. sea salt
2 Tbsp. sake

Mix the soup stock and water and bring them to a boil. Add the salt, cook this 20 minutes, then add the tofu and the watercress.

Boil it again, then add the beaten egg. As you add the egg, keep stirring the soup with a ladle so that the egg cooks in small pieces.

Add the sake and boil it once again. Serve it hot.

Fruit Cake 334.

3 cups apple juice, home-made
5 cups cold water
3 cups currants
2 cups dates, sliced
3 cups apricots
½ cup dried cherries
2 cups pecans
2 cups prunes
3 cups tangerine juice
10 cups whole wheat pastry flour
1 tsp. sea salt
½ cup oil
⅔ cup boiling water

Grate apples and squeeze them through a cotton cloth.

Mix the apple juice and 3 cups of cold water, then add the dates and apricots. Bring this to a boil and cook covered on a low flame for 4 hours.

Place the prunes and cherries in 2 cups of cold water. Cook them 20 minutes, cool them and remove the pits.

Roast the pecans in a frying pan until they are slightly brown. Add the nuts, prunes and cherries to the apricots and dates. Cook this mixture for 4 hours, covered.

Let this cool completely. Mix in the tangerine juice, place in a ceramic crock and let it sit for 10 days in a cool place. Be sure to stir it daily. Fermentation will begin and the smell will change somewhat.

Sift the flour and salt together. Mix the oil with ⅔ cup of boiling water; add the fruit mixture and the sifted flour to this, making a soft, smooth batter. (If you have time, place this in an oiled bowl, cover with a cloth or lid and let it sit for 2 or 3 days in a cool place.)

Oil and flour bread pans and place the mixture in the pans. Bake the cakes at 250° - 275° for 2 - 3 hours until they test dry with a bamboo skewer. While baking them, place a pan of cold water in the oven to keep the desired humidity. This helps them bake evenly and prevents the tops of the cakes from browning too fast.

Cool and wrap them in clean cotton cloths that have been soaked in brandy or sherry. Wrap this in aluminum foil to prevent evaporation of the moisture. Unwrap and re-saturate the cloths every few days.

Gluten Starch Pudding 335.

4 cups starch water (see 87.)
1 cup currants or raisins (if using raisins, chop them)
½ cup walnuts, chopped
1 tsp. sea salt
1 tsp. cinnamon

This pudding is made with gluten water (87.). Mix all the ingredients together and let them sit for 1 hour.

Heat and oil a cookie sheet or bread pan. Dust it with corn meal, then bake the pudding in a 350° oven for 1 hour; or, steam it in a bread pan for 40 minutes or until it becomes transparent.

Serve it cold.

Variation: Into this pudding you can also mix one cup of sliced peaches, apples, pears or other seasonal fruits.

Suggestions for Cooking

When using oil to saute vegetables for miso soup or nitsuke vegetable dishes, I use sesame oil. For pan-frying, bread baking or deep-frying, I use corn oil. In both cases these should be good quality, cold-pressed oils from a health food store.

For miso, I recommend barley (mugi) miso.

Brown rice should be short grain rice. This is the most balanced.

Tamari should be the highest quality. Lima soy sauce, available from Chico-San, is my recommendation.

Salt should be unrefined sea salt containing trace minerals.

For cooking utensils, use all heavy pots and pans such as cast iron, enamel ware or stainless steel. Avoid aluminum. I use a stainless steel pressure cooker.

Eggs should be fertile and organic. The same with all dairy products, when used. Toxic accumulation is greater in commercially raised animal products than in commercially grown grains and vegetables.

Spring water or well-water is preferable whenever possible.

Tofu, if purchased, should be prepared naturally with nigari instead of chemical agents.

Guide to Festive Meals

New Year's - January 1
GOMF Anniversary - January 21
Mari's Birthday - January 27
Chinese New Year - February 17
Girls' Day – March 3
Cornellia's Birthday – March 31
Jiro's Birthday – April 14
George Ohsawa Memorial Service – April 15
Boys' Day Eve – May 4
Michio Kushi Dinner – May 21
GOMF Director's Meeting – May 31
July 4th Ceremony – July 4
Non-macrobiotic Parents' Dinner – September 12
Wedding – September 16
Herman's Birthday – September 27
George Ohsawa's Birthday – October 17
Thanksgiving – November 22
Christmas – December 25

Menus

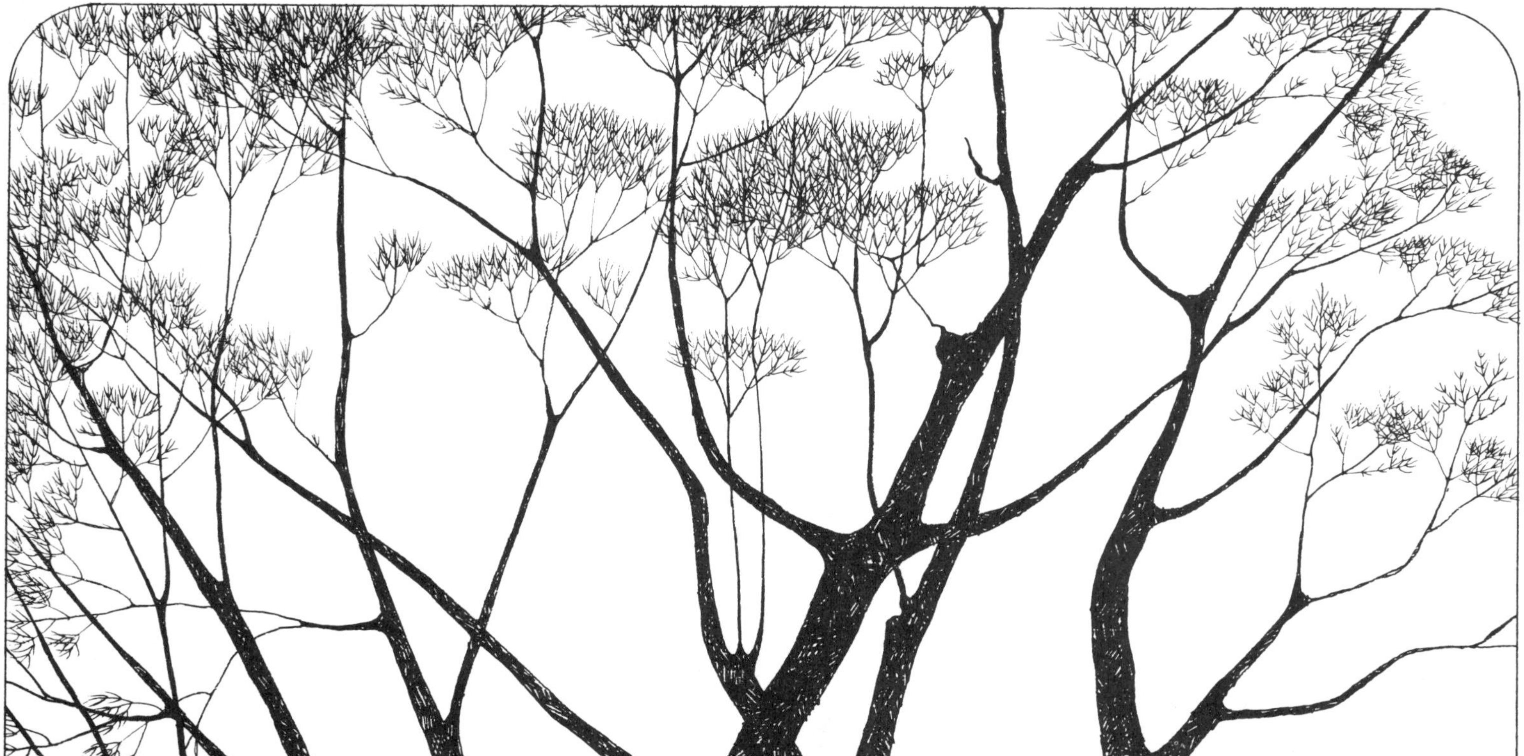

January

Breakfast		Dinner
1a. Azuki bean rice 1b. Pressure-cooked brown rice 1c. Brown rice, boiled 2A. Sweet brown rice mochi 2B. Steamed mochi 2C. Mugwort mochi 2a. Mochi soup 2b. Azuki bean mochi 2c. Walnut mochi 2d. Baked mochi with kinako 2e. Baked mochi with nori 3. Lotus root, burdock, carrot, konnyaku nishime 4. Kombu, age, albi nishime 5. Black bean nishime 6. Daikon, carrot salad 7. Yam - chestnut kinton 8. Amasake 8a. Amasake kanten 9. Tazukuri with yinnie syrup 10. Baked fish with salt 11. Rolled egg 12. Bancha (twig) tea	**Monday, January 1**	*Special Day – one meal only.*
2a. Mochi soup 1b. Pressure-cooked brown rice 3. Vegetable nishime 13. Natto with pickled daikon leaves 14,15. Daikon, Chinese cabbage nuka pickles	**Tuesday, January 2**	1b. Pressure-cooked brown rice 16,64. Buckwheat noodles with clear soup *with* Home-made age 17. Chick pea sauce 232. Dill pickles
18. Turnip, onion, carrot miso soup 1b. Pressure-cooked brown rice 19. Collard green, onion, carrot, celery nitsuke 5. Black bean nishime 14,15. Daikon, Chinese cabbage nuka pickles	**Wednesday, January 3**	1b. Pressure-cooked brown rice 20. Mackerel with ginger miso 21a,b. Tossed salad with dressing 15. Chinese cabbage nuka pickles 334. Fruit cake

Breakfast		Dinner
18. Turnip, onion, carrot miso soup 1b. Pressure-cooked brown rice 22a. Assorted vegetable tempura 23. Grated daikon 15. Chinese cabbage nuka pickles	**Thursday, January 4**	1b. Pressure-cooked brown rice 24,25. Kasha *with* Sesame sauce 26. Boiled beets 27. Azuki chestnut kanten
28. Wakame, onion, carrot miso soup 1b. Pressure-cooked brown rice 3. Leftover New Year's vegetables 14,15. Daikon, Chinese cabbage nuka pickles	**Friday, January 5**	1b. Pressure-cooked brown rice 29. Pan-fried whole wheat spaghetti 30. Nori nitsuke 31. Apple pie 15. Chinese cabbage nuka pickles
28. Wakame, onion, carrot miso soup 1b. Pressure-cooked brown rice 32. Kidney beans with miso 14,15. Daikon, Chinese cabbage nuka pickles	**Saturday, January 6**	1b. Pressure-cooked brown rice 33. Vegetable stew with sake 5. Black bean nishime 15. Chinese cabbage nuka pickles
28. Wakame, onion, carrot miso soup 1b. Pressure-cooked brown rice 34. Winter squash and onion nitsuke 14,15. Daikon, Chinese cabbage nuka pickles	**Sunday, January 7**	1b. Pressure-cooked brown rice 29. Whole wheat spaghetti (leftover) 30. Nori nitsuke (leftover) 14,15. Daikon, cabbage nuka pickles
28. Wakame, onion, carrot miso soup 1b. Pressure-cooked brown rice 35. Onion miso 14. Daikon nuka pickles	**Monday, January 8**	1b. Pressure-cooked brown rice 29. Pan-fried spaghetti with vegetables 32,34. Kidney beans with miso *mixed with* Winter squash and onion miso 15. Chinese cabbage nuka pickles
18,2C. Turnip, onion, daikon, carrot miso soup *with* Mugwort mochi 1b. Pressure-cooked brown rice 36. Vegetable gratin 14,15. Daikon, Chinese cabbage nuka pickles	**Tuesday, January 9**	1b. Pressure-cooked brown rice 38,37a. Kasha croquettes *with* Onion sake bechamel sauce 66,37. Boiled broccoli *with* Bechamel sauce 39. Lettuce goma ai 15. Chinese cabbage nuka pickles

Breakfast		*Dinner*
18, 2C. Turnip, daikon, onion, carrot miso soup *with* Mugwort mochi 1b. Pressure-cooked brown rice 32,5. Kidney beans (leftover) *with* Black bean nishime 14. Daikon nuka pickles	**Wednesday, January 10**	40. Russian soup with quail bone 41. Baked rice 30. Nori nitsuke 42. Prune kanten 15. Chinese cabbage nuka pickles
28. Wakame, leek, Chinese cabbage miso soup 1b. Pressure-cooked brown rice 43. Burdock, carrot, lotus root kinpira 14,15. Daikon, Chinese cabbage nuka pickles	**Thursday, January 11**	1b. Pressure-cooked brown rice 24,25. Kasha *with* Tahini sauce 44. Boiled Chinese cabbage 45. Rice loaf 14,15. Daikon, Chinese cabbage nuka pickles
18. Onion, Chinese cabbage, carrot, cabbage miso soup 1b. Pressure-cooked brown rice 46. Burdock, lotus root, carrot oily miso 14,15. Daikon, Chinese cabbage nuka pickles	**Friday, January 12**	1b. Pressure-cooked brown rice 47. Cauliflower with kuzu sauce 48. Parsnip and celery nitsuke 14,15. Daikon, Chinese cabbage nuka pickles
18. Onion, Chinese cabbage, carrot, cabbage miso soup 1b. Pressure-cooked brown rice 49. Rice cream 14. Daikon nuka pickles	**Saturday, January 13**	1b. Pressure-cooked brown rice 50. Millet with chick pea sauce 51. Hijiki with lotus root 15. Chinese cabbage nuka pickles
52. Vegetable ojiya 34. Winter squash and onion nitsuke 14. Daikon nuka pickles	**Sunday, January 14**	1b. Pressure-cooked brown rice 53. Udon with clear soup (quail-bone stock) 54. Broccoli nitsuke 15. Chinese cabbage nuka pickles
18. Onion, Chinese cabbage, carrot miso soup 1a. Azuki bean rice 49. Rice cream 55. Cabbage nitsuke 14,15. Daikon, Chinese cabbage nuka pickles	**Monday, January 15**	1b. Pressure-cooked brown rice 56. Garlic bread 50. Chick pea sauce (leftover) 30. Nori nitsuke (leftover) 14,15. Daikon, Chinese cabbage nuka pickles

Breakfast		Dinner
52. Vegetable ojiya 43. Burdock, carrot, lotus root kinpira 14,15. Daikon, Chinese cabbage nuka pickles	**Tuesday, January 16**	*Cooking Class* 28. Wakame, onion miso soup 1b. Pressure-cooked brown rice 57. Carrot and sesame seed nitsuke 58. French bread 59. Chinese cabbage pressed salad
18. Onion, turnip, carrot miso soup 1b. Pressure-cooked brown rice 34. Winter squash and onion nitsuke 15. Chinese cabbage nuka pickles	**Wednesday, January 17**	62. Sakura rice 60. Vegetable oden 61. Green pea nitsuke 14,15. Daikon, Chinese cabbage nuka pickles
18. Onion, turnip, cabbage, carrot miso soup 1b. Pressure-cooked brown rice 55. Cabbage nitsuke 15. Chinese cabbage nuka pickles	**Thursday, January 18**	1b. Pressure-cooked brown rice 24,53. Kasha (leftover) *mixed with* Udon (leftover) 61,17. Green pea nitsuke *with* Chick pea sauce 14,15. Daikon, Chinese cabbage nuka pickles
18. Onion, turnip, cabbage, carrot miso soup 1b. Pressure-cooked brown rice 63,64. Collard green *with* Home-made age 14,15. Daikon, Chinese cabbage nuka pickles	**Friday, January 19**	1b. Pressure-cooked brown rice 65,37. Millet croquettes *with* Bechamel sauce 66. Mustard green ohitashi with kirigoma 15. Chinese cabbage nuka pickles
18. Onion, turnip, cabbage, carrot miso soup 1b. Pressure-cooked brown rice 55. Cabbage nitsuke 14,15. Daikon, Chinese cabbage nuka pickles	**Saturday, January 20**	1b. Pressure-cooked brown rice 60. Oden (leftover) 66. Mustard green ohitashi 15. Chinese cabbage nuka pickles
GOMF Anniversary Dinner 62. Sakura rice with sesame seeds 11. Rolled egg 67. Burdock, carrot roll 267. Musubi kombu 9. Tazukuri with yinnie syrup 6. Daikon, carrot salad 7. Yam kinton 8a. Amasake kanten	**Sunday, January 21**	*Anniversary dinner continued – served as one meal at noon* 68. Karinto 14. Daikon nuka pickles Rice cakes and corn chips from Chico-San Fresh tangerines

Breakfast		Dinner
18. Scallion miso soup 1b. Pressure-cooked brown rice 55. Cabbage nitsuke 14,15. Daikon, Chinese cabbage nuka pickles	**Monday, January 22**	1b. Pressure-cooked brown rice 16. Buckwheat noodles with clear soup 5. Black bean nishime 6. Daikon and carrot salad
28. Wakame, onion, carrot miso soup 1b. Pressure-cooked brown rice 60. Oden (leftover) 5. Black bean nishime 14,15. Daikon, Chinese cabbage nuka pickles	**Tuesday, January 23**	*Cooking Class* 1b. Pressure-cooked brown rice 69. Split pea and macaroni potage 35. Onion miso 70. Sauteed cabbage and bean sprouts 8b. Amasake kanten
28. Wakame, onion, carrot miso soup 1b. Pressure-cooked brown rice 63. Collard green nitsuke 46. Burdock, onion, carrot with oily miso 14,15. Daikon, Chinese cabbage nuka pickles	**Wednesday, January 24**	1b. Pressure-cooked brown rice 29. Pan-fried spaghetti 21a,b. Tossed salad *with* dressing 15. Chinese cabbage nuka pickles
28. Wakame, onion, carrot miso soup 1b. Pressure-cooked brown rice 71. Azuki winter squash nitsuke 14,15. Daikon, Chinese cabbage nuka pickles	**Thursday, January 25**	1b. Pressure-cooked brown rice 69. Split pea and macaroni potage (leftover) 72. Kombu, nori nitsuke 31. Apple pie 14,15. Daikon, Chinese cabbage nuka pickles
28,69. Wakame, onion, carrot miso soup *mixed with* Split pea macaroni soup 1b. Pressure-cooked brown rice 13. Natto with pickled daikon leaves 60,63. Vegetable oden *mixed with* Collard green nitsuke 14,15. Daikon, Chinese cabbage nuka pickles	**Friday, January 26**	1b. Pressure-cooked brown rice 74. Uosuki 75. Northern white beans with white miso 31. Apple pie 14,15. Daikon, Chinese cabbage nuka pickles

Breakfast		*Dinner*
18. Daikon, burdock, carrot miso soup 1b. Pressure-cooked brown rice 35. Onion miso 267. Musubi kombu 14,15. Daikon, Chinese cabbage nuka pickles	**Saturday, January 27**	*Mari's Birthday Party* 41. Baked rice 76,76a. Macaroni salad *with* Mayonnaise 77,79. Mashed potatoes *with* Gravy 78. Fried chicken 21a,b. Tossed salad *with* Dressing 80a. Clear soup with tofu and shingiku 81. White buns 82. Amasake cake with frosting
18. Daikon, burdock, carrot miso soup 1b. Pressure-cooked brown rice 83. Waffles with maple syrup, butter and honey 35. Onion miso 14,15. Daikon, Chinese cabbage nuka pickles	**Sunday, January 28**	1b. Pressure-cooked brown rice 29,79. Fried spaghetti *with* Gravy 21a. Tossed salad 15. Chinese cabbage nuka pickles
18,79. Daikon, burdock, carrot miso soup *mixed with* Gravy 1b. Pressure-cooked brown rice 2d. Baked mochi with kinako 71,61,75. Azuki-squash, Green pea *and* Northern white bean nitsuke, all mixed 15. Chinese cabbage nuka pickles	**Monday, January 29**	1b. Pressure-cooked brown rice 84,79,37. Noodle burger *with* Gravy *and* Bechamel sauce, parsley garnish 85. Chinese cabbage, onion, carrot nitsuke 14,15. Daikon, Chinese cabbage nuka pickles
18,2C. Onion, Chinese cabbage, carrot miso soup *with* Mugwort mochi 1b. Pressure-cooked brown rice 86. Fresh daikon nitsuke 67. Burdock roll (leftover) 14,15. Daikon, Chinese cabbage nuka pickles	**Tuesday, January 30**	1b. Pressure-cooked brown rice 80b. Tofu - scallion miso soup 87e. Gluten cutlets with vegetable kebabs 88. Fried saifun with lettuce 89. Daikon and daikon leaves pressed salad 90. Oatmeal cookies
18. Onion, Chinese cabbage, carrot miso soup 1b. Pressure-cooked brown rice 13. Natto with pickled daikon leaves 35. Onion miso 14,15. Daikon, Chinese cabbage nuka pickles	**Wednesday, January 31**	1b. Pressure-cooked brown rice 53. Clear soup with noodles 55. Cabbage, cauliflower nitsuke 14,15. Daikon, Chinese cabbage nuka pickles

February

Breakfast		Day	Dinner	
18.	Onion, Chinese cabbage, carrot miso soup	**Thursday, February 1**	1b.	Pressure-cooked brown rice
1a.	Azuki bean rice		91.	Saifun nitsuke
43.	Burdock, carrot kinpira		72.	Kombu, nori nitsuke
14.	Daikon nuka pickles		14,15.	Daikon, Chinese cabbage nuka pickles
28.	Wakame, onion, cabbage miso soup	**Friday, February 2**	1b.	Pressure-cooked brown rice
1b.	Pressure-cooked brown rice		29.	Pan-fried whole wheat spaghetti
92.	Mustard green and carrot with tempura		21a,b.	Tossed salad with dressing
83.	Waffles		93.	Halvah
14.	Daikon nuka pickles			
1b.	Pressure-cooked brown rice	**Saturday, February 3**	1b.	Pressure-cooked brown rice
36,87d.	Vegetable gratin *with* Gluten cutlets		95.	Pan-fried fish
51.	Hijiki, lotus root nitsuke		91.	Saifun nitsuke
94.	Muffins		15.	Chinese cabbage nuka pickles
14.	Daikon nuka pickles			
28.	Wakame miso soup	**Sunday, February 4**	1b.	Pressure-cooked brown rice
1b.	Pressure-cooked brown rice		53.	Clear soup with noodles
55.	Cabbage, cauliflower nitsuke		29.	Fried noodles (leftover)
15.	Chinese cabbage nuka pickles		21a,b.	Tossed salad (leftover)
28.	Wakame miso soup	**Monday, February 5**	1b.	Pressure-cooked brown rice
1b.	Pressure-cooked brown rice		37,87d.	Vegetable gratin *with* Gluten cutlets
96.	Rice kayu		51.	Hijiki with lotus root
97.	Scallion miso		15.	Chinese cabbage nuka pickles
98.	Mustard green pressed salad			
52.	Vegetable ojiya	**Tuesday, February 6**		*Cooking Class*
99.	Wheat cream		1b.	Pressure-cooked brown rice
43.	Burdock, carrot kinpira		16.	Buckwheat noodles with clear soup
14,15.	Daikon, Chinese cabbage nuka pickles		100.	Okara nitsuke
			98.	Mustard green pressed salad
			45.	Rice loaf
			93.	Halvah

Breakfast		Dinner
18. Cabbage, onion, carrot miso soup 1b. Pressure-cooked brown rice 99. Wheat cream 91. Saifun nitsuke 101. Sauteed mustard pickles 14,15. Daikon, Chinese cabbage nuka pickles	**Wednesday, February 7**	1b. Pressure-cooked brown rice 29. Pan-fried whole wheat spaghetti 56. Garlic bread 71. Kidney beans with yam nitsuke 14,15. Daikon, Chinese cabbage nuka pickles
18. Cabbage, onion, carrot miso soup 1b. Pressure-cooked brown rice 49. Rice cream 36. Vegetable gratin 98. Mustard pickles	**Thursday, February 8**	1b. Pressure-cooked brown rice 102. Buckwheat noodles gratin with kuzu sauce 48. Parsnip, celery nitsuke 14,15. Daikon, Chinese cabbage nuka pickles
18. Cabbage, onion, carrot miso soup 1b. Pressure-cooked brown rice 103. Vegetables with tahini sauce 30. Nori nitsuke 15. Chinese cabbage nuka pickles	**Friday, February 9**	1b. Pressure-cooked brown rice 87d. Gluten cutlets 104. Fresh daikon with lemon miso sauce 80,80b. Tofu - scallion miso soup *with* Home-made tofu 15. Chinese cabbage nuka pickles
52. Vegetable ojiya 36. Vegetable gratin 13. Natto with pickled daikon leaves 14,15. Daikon, Chinese cabbage nuka pickles	**Saturday, February 10**	1b. Pressure-cooked brown rice 105. Baked smelt 39. Lettuce goma ai 106. Buckwheat noodle burger 14. Daikon nuka pickles
18. Burdock, daikon, carrot miso soup 1b. Pressure-cooked brown rice 2d. Baked mochi with kinako 36. Vegetable gratin (leftover) 83. Waffles 15. Chinese cabbage nuka pickles	**Sunday, February 11**	1b. Pressure-cooked brown rice 53. Clear soup with udon 14,15. Daikon, Chinese cabbage nuka pickles
18. Burdock, daikon, carrot miso soup 1b. Pressure-cooked brown rice 2d. Baked mochi with kinako 32. Kidney beans with miso 14,15. Daikon, Chinese cabbage nuka pickles	**Monday, February 12**	1b. Pressure-cooked brown rice 107. Sauteed carrot with kidney beans 102. Buckwheat noodles with kuzu sauce 108. Squash cake 15. Chinese cabbage nuka pickles

Breakfast		Dinner
18. Burdock, daikon, carrot miso soup 1b. Pressure-cooked brown rice 2d. Baked mochi with kinako 63,64. Collard green *and* age nitsuke 14,15. Daikon, Chinese cabbage nuka pickles	**Tuesday, February 13**	*Cooking Class* 53. Clear soup with noodles 87d. Gluten cutlets 55. Cabbage nitsuke 41. Baked rice 109. Gomashio 31. Apple pie 15. Chinese cabbage nuka pickles
28. Wakame miso soup 1b. Pressure-cooked brown rice 32. Kidney beans (leftover) 97. Scallion miso 14,15. Daikon, Chinese cabbage nuka pickles	**Wednesday, February 14**	1b. Pressure-cooked brown rice 38,37a. Kasha croquettes *with* Bechamel sauce 48. Parsnip - celery nitsuke 31. Apple pie 14. Daikon nuka pickles
80b. Tofu - scallion miso soup 1a. Azuki bean rice 86. Fresh daikon nitsuke 14,15. Daikon, Chinese cabbage nuka pickles	**Thursday, February 15**	1b. Pressure-cooked brown rice 110. Vegetable stew 97. Scallion miso 31. Apple pie 15. Chinese cabbage nuka pickles
18. Turnip, onion, carrot miso soup 1b. Pressure-cooked brown rice 36. Vegetable gratin (leftover) 14,15. Daikon, Chinese cabbage nuka pickles	**Friday, February 16**	1b. Pressure-cooked brown rice 50. Millet with chick pea sauce 72. Kombu - nori nitsuke 56. Garlic bread 111. Chick pea spread 15. Chinese cabbage nuka pickles
18. Turnip, onion, carrot miso soup 1b. Pressure-cooked brown rice 55. Cabbage nitsuke 14,15. Daikon, Chinese cabbage nuka pickles	**Saturday, February 17**	*Chinese New Year Dinner* 1b. Pressure-cooked brown rice 112. Deep-fried fish with kuzu sauce 113. Egg foo yung 114. Saifun salad 115a. Egg drop soup 116. Tuna sashimi 117. Pineapple - apple open-face pie

Breakfast		*Dinner*
18. Miso soup (leftover) 1b. Pressure-cooked brown rice 86. Fresh daikon nitsuke (leftover) 15. Chinese cabbage nuka pickles	**Sunday, February 18**	1b. Pressure-cooked brown rice 66. Green vegetable ohitashi with bonita flakes 112. Deep-fried fish (leftover) 117. Pineapple - apple pie (leftover) 14. Daikon nuka pickles
18. Cabbage, onion, carrot miso soup 1b. Pressure-cooked brown rice 13. Natto with pickled daikon leaves 86. Fresh daikon nitsuke 15. Chinese cabbage nuka pickles	**Monday, February 19**	1b. Pressure-cooked brown rice 65,37. Millet croquettes *with* Bechamel sauce 14,15. Nuka pickles
18. Chinese cabbage, onion, carrot miso soup 1b. Pressure-cooked brown rice 50. Chick pea sauce (leftover) 66,76a. Ohitashi (leftover) *with* Mayonnaise and tamari soy sauce	**Tuesday, February 20**	*Cooking Class* 1b. Pressure-cooked brown rice 47. Cauliflower with kuzu sauce 30. Nori nitsuke 92. Halvah 15. Chinese cabbage nuka pickles
18. Daikon, onion, carrot miso soup 1b. Pressure-cooked brown rice 2e. Baked mochi with nori, soy sauce 2d. Baked mochi with amasake-kinako 54. Broccoli nitsuke 14,15. Daikon, Chinese cabbage nuka pickles	**Wednesday, February 21**	119. Fried rice 118. Baked squash with sesame sauce 66. Ohitashi with kirigoma 93. Halvah 14. Daikon nuka pickles
18. Turnip, onion, carrot miso soup 1b. Pressure-cooked brown rice 85. Chinese cabbage, onion, carrot nitsuke 14. Daikon, daikon leaves nuka pickles	**Thursday, February 22**	1b. Pressure-cooked brown rice 120. Tuna shish-kebab with barbeque sauce 21a,b. Tossed salad with dressing 121. White rice 14. Daikon nuka pickles
18. Leek, Chinese cabbage, carrot miso soup 1b. Pressure-cooked brown rice 54,86. Broccoli *and* Fresh daikon nitsuke mixed 15. Chinese cabbage, takana nuka pickles	**Friday, February 23**	1b. Pressure-cooked brown rice 22,122. Vegetable tempura *with* sauce 23. Grated daikon 123. Chinese cabbage roll 124. Apple crisp 15. Chinese cabbage nuka pickles

Breakfast		Dinner
18. Leek, Chinese cabbage, carrot miso soup 1b. Pressure-cooked brown rice 22. Tempura (leftover) 125,126. Rice balls *with* Shio kombu 15. Chinese cabbage nuka pickles	**Saturday, February 24**	*Dinner out.*
Gone to Chico.	**Sunday, February 25**	*Gone to Chico.*
18. Leek, cauliflower leaves, carrot miso soup 1b. Pressure-cooked brown rice 55. Cabbage nitsuke 14,15. Daikon, Chinese cabbage nuka pickles	**Monday, February 26**	119. Fried rice 53. Whole wheat spaghetti with broth 72. Nori - kombu nitsuke 15. Chinese cabbage nuka pickles
18. Leek, cauliflower leaves, carrot miso soup 1b. Pressure-cooked brown rice 19. Turnip, turnip leaves, onion, carrot nitsuke 14,15. Daikon, Chinese cabbage nuka pickles	**Tuesday, February 27**	*Cooking Class* 1b. Pressure-cooked brown rice 127. Squash potage with croutons 66. Chinese mustard green ohitashi 128. Pan-fried gyoza with lemon sauce 15. Chinese cabbage nuka pickles
28. Wakame, onion, carrot miso soup 1b. Pressure-cooked brown rice 92. New Zealand spinach, onion nitsuke 13. Natto with pickled daikon leaves 14,15. Daikon, Chinese cabbage nuka pickles	**Wednesday, February 28**	1b. Pressure-cooked brown rice 128. Pan-fried gyoza with lemon sauce 129. Clear soup with vegetables 15. Chinese cabbage nuka pickles

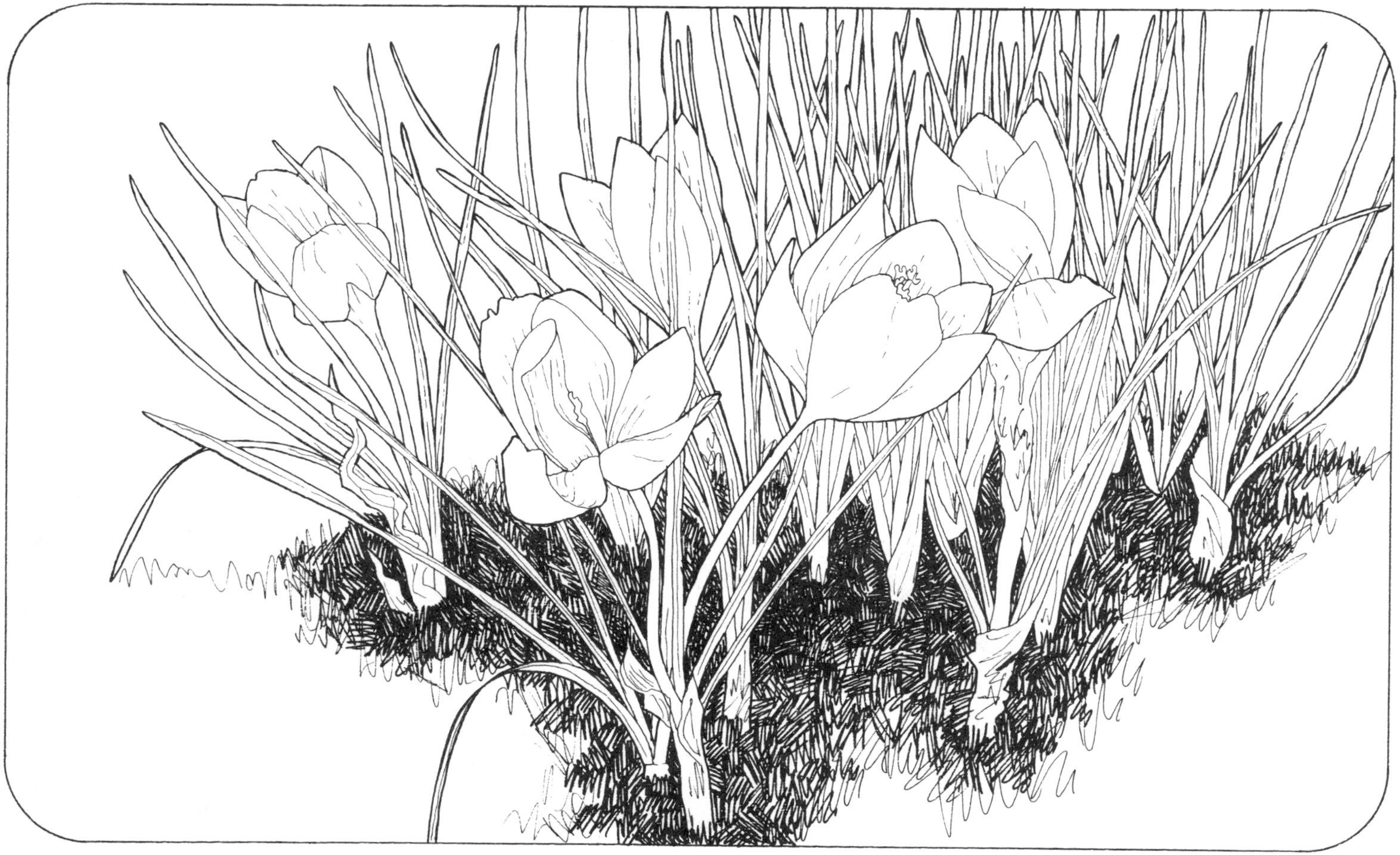

March

Breakfast			Dinner	
28.	Wakame, onion, carrot miso soup	**Thursday, March 1**	1b.	Pressure-cooked brown rice
1b.	Pressure-cooked brown rice		2a.	Brown rice mochi soup
118,55.	Baked squash and turnip (leftover) *mixed with* Cabbage nitsuke		2c.	Walnut mochi
14.	Turnip, turnip leaves nuka pickles		2b.	Azuki bean mochi
			2d.	Baked mochi with kinako
			91.	Saifun nitsuke
			14.	Daikon nuka pickles
28.	Wakame, onion, carrot miso soup	**Friday, March 2**	1b.	Pressure-cooked brown rice
1b.	Pressure-cooked brown rice		130.	Rice pie
63.	Collard green nitsuke		47.	Cauliflower with kuzu sauce
14,15.	Daikon, Chinese cabbage nuka pickles		15.	Chinese cabbage nuka pickles
18.	Chinese cabbage, onion, cauliflower leaves miso soup	**Saturday, March 3**		*Girls' Day*
1b.	Pressure-cooked brown rice		1b.	Pressure-cooked brown rice
131.	Wild scallion and egg nitsuke		2a.	Mochi soup
49.	Rice cream		2b,c,d.	Mochi (leftover)
14.	Daikon nuka pickles		91.	Saifun nitsuke
			132.	Amasake cake with yannoh frosting
			14,15.	Daikon, Chinese cabbage nuka pickles
18.	Chinese cabbage, onion, cauliflower leaves miso soup	**Sunday, March 4**	1b.	Pressure-cooked brown rice
1b.	Pressure-cooked brown rice		235.	Udon with clear soup
48.	Celery sticks nitsuke (similar)		91.	Saifun nitsuke (leftover)
14,15.	Daikon, Chinese cabbage nuka pickles		15.	Chinese cabbage nuka pickles
18.	Chinese cabbage, onion, cauliflower leaves miso soup	**Monday, March 5**	1b.	Pressure-cooked brown rice
1b.	Pressure-cooked brown rice		24,25.	Kasha *with* Sesame onion sauce
99.	Wheat cream		133.	Yam, carrot nitsuke
13.	Natto with pickled daikon leaves		15.	Chinese cabbage nuka pickles
91.	Saifun nitsuke (leftover)			
15.	Chinese cabbage nuka pickles			

Breakfast		Dinner
18. Cabbage, onion, carrot miso soup 1b. Pressure-cooked brown rice 54. Broccoli nitsuke 14,15. Daikon, Chinese cabbage nuka pickles	**Tuesday, March 6**	*Cooking Class* 134. Gomoku rice 18. Turnip, turnip leaves, onion, carrot miso soup 123. Chinese cabbage roll 135. Amasake yeasted doughnuts
18. Turnip, turnip leaves, onion, carrot miso soup 1b. Pressure-cooked brown rice 63. Mustard green, age, carrot nitsuke 99. Wheat cream 14,15. Daikon, Chinese cabbage nuka pickles	**Wednesday, March 7**	1b. Pressure-cooked brown rice 107. Kidney beans with carrot 39. Lettuce goma ai 56. Garlic bread 14,15. Chinese cabbage, daikon nuka pickles
18,2c. Miso soup (leftover) with scallions *and* Mugwort mochi 1b. Pressure-cooked brown rice 63. Vegetable nitsuke (leftover) 97. Scallion, scallion roots miso 14. Daikon nuka pickles	**Thursday, March 8**	1b. Pressure-cooked brown rice 38. Kasha croquettes dusted with sweet rice flour 37. Bechamel sauce 48. Parsnip - celery nitsuke 98. Mustard green pressed salad
18. Turnip, turnip leaves, onion miso soup 1b. Pressure-cooked brown rice 19. Collard green, onion, carrot nitsuke 137. Mustard green nuka pickles	**Friday, March 9**	1b. Pressure-cooked brown rice 69. Split pea macaroni soup 138. Vegetable kebabs with lemon sauce 98. Mustard green pressed salad 14. Daikon nuka pickles
18. Beet, beet top, leek, carrot miso soup 1b. Pressure-cooked brown rice 49. Rice cream 13. Natto with pickled daikon leaves 139. Dandelion leaves and root, cabbage nitsuke 15,137. Chinese cabbage, mustard green nuka pickles	**Saturday, March 10**	1b. Pressure-cooked brown rice 120. Chicken and turkey giblet kebabs with barbecue sauce 26. Cooked beet and beet tops with umeboshi 90. Oatmeal cookies 15. Chinese cabbage nuka pickles Fresh tangerines

Breakfast		*Dinner*
18. Turnip top, onion, leek, carrot miso soup 1b. Pressure-cooked brown rice 69,107. Split pea soup (leftover) *mixed with* Kidney beans (leftover) 19. Collard green and onion nitsuke (leftover) 14,15. Daikon, Chinese cabbage nuka pickles	**Sunday, March 11**	1b. Pressure-cooked brown rice 38,37. Kasha croquettes (leftover) *with* Bechamel sauce 21a,76a. Tossed salad *with* Mayonnaise sauce 48. Parsnip - celery nitsuke (leftover) 90. Oatmeal cookies
2d. Burdock, daikon, carrot mochi soup 1b. Pressure-cooked brown rice 36,37. Vegetable gratin (all leftover nitsuke, mixed) *with* Bechamel sauce 14,15. Daikon, Chinese cabbage nuka pickles	**Monday, March 12**	1b. Pressure-cooked brown rice 118. Baked Hokkaido pumpkin with onion sesame sauce 140. Dried daikon nitsuke 15. Chinese cabbage nuka pickles
2a. Mochi soup 1b. Pressure-cooked brown rice 35. Onion miso 19. Green vegetable nitsuke 141. Condiment pickles 14. Daikon nuka pickles	**Tuesday, March 13**	*Cooking Class* 28. Wakame, onion, carrot miso soup 1b. Pressure-cooked brown rice 50. Millet with chick pea sauce 140. Dried daikon nitsuke 98. Mustard green pressed salad 142. Baked apples
28. Wakame, onion, carrot miso soup 1b. Pressure-cooked brown rice 49. Rice cream 63. Green vegetable nitsuke 14,15. Daikon, Chinese cabbage nuka pickles	**Wednesday, March 14**	1b. Pressure-cooked brown rice 29. Pan-fried whole wheat spaghetti 80. Home-made tofu with bonita flakes 15. Chinese cabbage nuka pickles 124. Apple crisp
1a. Azuki bean rice 28. Wakame, onion, cabbage miso soup 54. Broccoli nitsuke 14,15. Daikon, Chinese cabbage nuka pickles	**Thursday, March 15**	1b. Pressure-cooked brown rice 24,25. Kasha *with* Sesame onion sauce 21a,143. Tossed salad *with* Umeboshi dressing 124. Apple crisp
28. Wakame, onion, cabbage miso soup 1b. Pressure-cooked brown rice 99. Wheat cream 100. Okara nitsuke 14,15. Daikon, Chinese cabbage nuka pickles	**Friday, March 16**	1b. Pressure-cooked brown rice 40. Russian soup with chicken stock 58. French bread (home-made) 140. Dried daikon nitsuke 137. Celery nuka pickles 144. Squash and dried fruit kanten

Breakfast		Dinner
18. Chinese cabbage, onion, cabbage, beet, carrot miso soup 1b. Pressure-cooked brown rice 99. Wheat cream 51. Hijiki, lotus root nitsuke 137. Cabbage, celery nuka pickles	**Saturday, March 17**	*Dinner out.*
Picnic 145. Sweet rice and azuki beans 146. Norimake sushi 147. Piroshki 132. Amasake cake 14. Daikon nuka pickles	**Sunday, March 18**	18. Vegetable miso soup 1b. Pressure-cooked brown rice 146. Norimake sushi (leftover) 147. Piroshki (leftover) 144. Squash and dried fruit kanten 15. Chinese cabbage nuka pickles
18. Cabbage, onion, carrot miso soup 1b. Pressure-cooked brown rice 99. Wheat cream 146. Steamed norimake sushi 66. Mustard green ohitashi with bonita 14,15. Daikon, Chinese cabbage nuka pickles	**Monday, March 19**	1b. Pressure-cooked brown rice 29. Pan-fried whole wheat spaghetti 148. Hijiki, nori nitsuke 145. Sweet rice and azuki beans (leftover) 124. Apple crisp 144. Squash and dried fruit kanten 14. Daikon nuka pickles
18,2C. Miso soup *with* Mugwort mochi 1b. Pressure-cooked brown rice 50,147. Chick pea sauce (leftover) *mixed with* Piroshki filling 140. Dried daikon nitsuke 14,15. Daikon, Chinese cabbage nuka pickles	**Tuesday, March 20**	*Cooking Class* 149. Ohagi - sweet rice ball with topping: green pea, brown sesame seeds, nori 36. Vegetable gratin 80a. Clear soup with tofu, shingiku 137. Celery nuka pickles
28. Cabbage, turnip, daikon, wakame miso soup 134,100. Gomoku rice *mixed with* Okara (leftover) 149. Ohagi (leftover) 99. Wheat cream 14,15. Daikon, Chinese cabbage nuka pickles	**Wednesday, March 21**	1b. Pressure-cooked brown rice 65,37. Millet croquettes *with* Bechamel sauce 66. Swiss chard ohitashi with kirigoma and bonita flakes 14. Daikon nuka pickles

Breakfast		Dinner
28. Cabbage, turnip, daikon, wakame miso soup 1b. Pressure-cooked brown rice 36,66. Vegetable gratin (leftover) *mixed with* Swiss chard ohitashi 13. Natto with pickled daikon leaves 14,15. Daikon, Chinese cabbage nuka pickles	**Thursday, March 22**	1b. Pressure-cooked brown rice 40,36. Russian soup (leftover) *mixed with* Vegetable gratin 150. Parsnip, yam nitsuke 14,15. Daikon, cabbage nuka pickles
18. Cauliflower leaves, cabbage, onion, turnip top, carrot miso soup 1b. Pressure-cooked brown rice 49. Rice cream 54. Broccoli nitsuke 14. Daikon nuka pickles	**Friday, March 23**	1b. Pressure-cooked brown rice 151. Stuffed cabbage with white sauce 97. Scallion miso 94,149. Muffins *with* Green pea filling 98. Mustard green pressed salad
18. Miso soup (leftover) 1b. Pressure-cooked brown rice 19. Collard green, onion, carrot nitsuke 83,152. Waffles *with* Home-made apple butter 97. Scallion miso 15. Chinese cabbage nuka pickles	**Saturday, March 24**	*Dinner Out.*
Gone for entire day.	**Sunday, March 25**	*Gone for entire day.*
28. Wakame, onion, cabbage, carrot miso soup 1b. Pressure-cooked brown rice 19. Collard green, onion, carrot nitsuke 97. Scallion miso 14,15. Daikon, Chinese cabbage nuka pickles	**Monday, March 26**	1b. Pressure-cooked brown rice 110. Vegetable stew 65,37. Millet croquettes *with* Bechamel sauce 30. Nori nitsuke 153. Rye bread

Breakfast		Dinner
28. Wakame, vegetable miso soup 1b. Pressure-cooked brown rice 49. Rice cream 86. Fresh daikon nitsuke 15. Chinese cabbage nuka pickles	**Tuesday, March 27**	*Cooking Class* 1b. Pressure-cooked brown rice 154. Vegetables with macaroni 146. Norimake sushi 75. Northern white beans with white rice miso 153. Rye bread 152. Home-made apple butter 15. Cabbage nuka pickles
28. Wakame, onion, cabbage, carrot miso soup 1b. Pressure-cooked brown rice 155. Burdock, onion, carrot fritters 14,15. Daikon, Chinese cabbage nuka pickles	**Wednesday, March 28**	1b. Pressure-cooked brown rice 64. Home-made age 110. Vegetable stew 66. Mustard green ohitashi with kirigoma and bonita flakes 121. White rice
18. Leek, mustard green, onion, carrot miso soup 1b. Pressure-cooked brown rice 13. Natto with pickled daikon leaves 19. Vegetable nitsuke (leftover) 14,15. Daikon, Chinese cabbage nuka pickles	**Thursday, March 29**	1b. Pressure-cooked brown rice 47. Cauliflower with kuzu sauce 30. Nori nitsuke 93. Halvah 15. Cabbage nuka pickles
18. Leek, mustard green, onion, carrot miso soup 1b. Pressure-cooked brown rice 71. Azuki squash nitsuke 14,15. Daikon, Chinese cabbage nuka pickles	**Friday, March 30**	1b. Pressure-cooked brown rice 87e. Gluten kebabs 21a. Tossed salad 93. Halvah
18. Leek, mustard green, onion, carrot miso soup 1b. Pressure-cooked brown rice 156. Horsetail nitsuke 14. Daikon nuka pickles	**Saturday, March 31**	*Cornellia's Birthday Party* 134. Gomoku rice 129. Clear party soup with vegetables 44. Chinese cabbage ohitashi 2C. Mugwort mochi 2d. Kinako mochi with amasake 98. Mustard green pressed salad 157. Eggplant mustard pickles

April

Breakfast		Dinner
134. Gomoku rice ball (leftover) 158. Sake-kasu cucumber pickles 14. Daikon nuka pickles Peanut butter sandwich	**Sunday, April 1**	1b. Pressure-cooked brown rice 53. Clear soup with noodles 15. Chinese cabbage nuka pickles
1a. Azuki bean rice 80b. Tofu, watercress miso soup 110. Vegetable stew with watercress (leftover) 156. Horsetail nitsuke (leftover) 14,15. Daikon, Chinese cabbage nuka pickles	**Monday, April 2**	1b. Pressure-cooked brown rice 91. Saifun nitsuke 72. Nori, kombu nitsuke 45. Rice loaf 14,15. Daikon, cabbage nuka pickles
18. Chinese cabbage, onion, carrot miso soup 1b. Pressure-cooked brown rice 54. Broccoli nitsuke 14,15. Daikon, Chinese cabbage nuka pickles	**Tuesday, April 3**	*Cooking Class* 1b. Pressure-cooked brown rice 159. Koi-koku (carp soup) 70. Sauteed cabbage and bean sprouts with onion and celery 142. Baked apple 15. Chinese cabbage nuka pickles
159,49. Koi-koku (leftover) *mixed with* Rice cream 1b. Pressure-cooked brown rice 91. Saifun nitsuke (leftover) 71. Azuki squash nitsuke 14,15. Daikon, Chinese cabbage nuka pickles	**Wednesday, April 4**	96. Rice kayu 160a. Whole wheat noodle salad 150. Yam, parsnip nitsuke with celery 137. Cabbage, turnip nuka pickle 142. Baked apple
18. Beet, onion, cabbage, carrot miso soup 1b. Pressure-cooked brown rice 13. Natto with pickled daikon leaves 140,87d. Dried daikon nitsuke (leftover) *with* Gluten cutlets 15. Chinese cabbage nuka pickles	**Thursday, April 5**	1b. Pressure-cooked brown rice 29. Pan-fried whole wheat spaghetti 26. Cooked beets 160a. Noodle salad (leftover) 161. Amasake cake with fruit and nuts 14. Daikon nuka pickles

Breakfast		Dinner
18. Beet, onion, cabbage, carrot, watercress miso soup 1b. Pressure-cooked brown rice 19. Collard green, onion, carrot nitsuke 13. Natto with pickled daikon leaves 14,15. Daikon, Chinese cabbage nuka pickles	**Friday, April 6**	1b. Pressure-cooked brown rice 47. Cauliflower with kuzu sauce with seitan 61. Green pea - onion nitsuke 161. Amasake cake 15. Chinese cabbage nuka pickles
96. Rice kayu 97. Scallion miso 140. Dried daikon nitsuke (leftover) 14,15. Daikon, Chinese cabbage nuka pickles	**Saturday, April 7**	162. Seitan goma rice 58. French bread 47. Cauliflower with kuzu sauce (leftover) 15. Chinese cabbage nuka pickles
Breakfast Out.	**Sunday, April 8**	1b. Pressure-cooked brown rice 29. Fried noodles (leftover) 150. Yam, parsnip nitsuke 163. Sauteed onion, potato, green pepper 161. Amasake cake 15. Chinese cabbage nuka pickles
28. Wakame, onion, cabbage, carrot miso soup 1b. Pressure-cooked brown rice 49. Rice cream 19. Collard green nitsuke (leftover) 13. Natto with pickled daikon leaves 141. Condiment pickles	**Monday, April 9**	1b. Pressure-cooked brown rice 164,37. Noodle croquettes *with* Bechamel sauce 61. Green pea nitsuke with onion 15. Chinese cabbage nuka pickles
28. Wakame, onion, cabbage, carrot miso soup 1b. Pressure-cooked brown rice 36. Vegetable gratin (leftover nitsuke) 64. Home-made age 23. Grated daikon and carrot 15. Chinese cabbage nuka pickles	**Tuesday, April 10**	*Cooking Class* 1b. Pressure-cooked brown rice 120. Fresh tuna shish-kebab with barbecue sauce 80b. Tofu - scallion miso soup 165. Raisin cake 15. Chinese cabbage nuka pickles

Breakfast		*Dinner*
18. Turnip, onion, carrot miso soup 1b. Pressure-cooked brown rice 13. Natto with pickled daikon leaves 30. Nori nitsuke 163. Sauteed vegetables (leftover) 14. Daikon nuka pickles	**Wednesday, April 11**	*Dinner Out.*
18,2C. Turnip, onion, cabbage, carrot miso soup *with* Mugwort mochi 1b. Pressure-cooked brown rice 19. Collard green, onion, carrot, celery nitsuke 14,15. Daikon, Chinese cabbage nuka pickles	**Thursday, April 12**	1b. Pressure-cooked brown rice 24,25. Kasha *with* Sesame onion sauce 309. Steamed cabbage 132. Amasake cake 14. Daikon nuka pickles
18. Squash, onion, scallion, scallion root miso soup 1b. Pressure-cooked brown rice 54. Broccoli nitsuke 14,15. Daikon, Chinese cabbage nuka pickles	**Friday, April 13**	1b. Pressure-cooked brown rice 50. Millet with chick pea sauce 66. Swiss chard, shingiku ohitashi 15. Chinese cabbage nuka pickles
18. Squash, onion, scallion, scallion root miso soup 1b. Pressure-cooked brown rice 140. Dried daikon nitsuke 15. Chinese cabbage nuka pickles	**Saturday, April 14**	*Jiro's Birthday Dinner* 166a, Roast wild duck with stuffing (similar) *with* 166b. Gravy 167. Sesame spaghetti with oyster sauce 41. Baked rice 168. Baked potato 21a. Tossed salad 165. Raisin cake 169. Fruit punch
1b. Pressure-cooked brown rice 171. Millet kayu 140,22c. Dried daikon nitsuke (leftover) *with* Tempura crumbs 97. Scallion miso 98. Mustard green pressed salad	**Sunday, April 15**	*George Ohsawa Memorial Service at Gedatsu Church* – early afternoon 149. Ohagi, sesame seed 149. Ohagi, azuki bean (similar 2b.) Corn chips *Dinner listing – next page*

Breakfast		*Dinner*
	Sunday, April 15 *(continued)*	149. Ohagi (leftover) 170. Rice bread 165. Birthday cake 14. Daikon nuka pickles
Mirimichi Camp begins.	**Monday, April 16**	28. Wakame, leek, carrot miso soup 1b. Pressure-cooked brown rice 149. Ohagi (leftover) 92. Mustard green nitsuke (similar) 172. Whole wheat flour tortillas 173. Horsetail - onion roll 174. Raisin roll
28,92. Miso soup (leftover) *with* Mustard green nitsuke (leftover) 1b. Pressure-cooked brown rice 175. Broccoli, mustard green nitsuke 14. Daikon nuka pickles	**Tuesday, April 17**	*Tea Time* 45,152. Rice loaf *with* Apple butter *Dinner* 1b. Pressure-cooked brown rice 128. Pan-fried gyoza 176. Lentil soup 21a. Tossed salad
177. Daikon, onion, cabbage, carrot miso soup with buchwheat dumplings 1b. Pressure-cooked brown rice 63. Collard green nitsuke 14. Daikon nuka pickles 21a. Salad (leftover)	**Wednesday, April 18**	*Tea Time* 178. Baked sweet potatoes *Dinner* 1b. Pressure-cooked brown rice 47. Cauliflower with kuzu sauce 30. Nori nitsuke 135. Amasake doughnuts 14. Daikon nuka pickles

Breakfast		*Dinner*
96. Rice kayu 47. Kuzu sauce (leftover) 97. Scallion miso 179. Bracken, onion, carrot, chirimen iriko nitsuke 137. Cabbage, celery nuka pickles	**Thursday, April 19**	*Picnic* 1b. Pressure-cooked brown rice 178. Sweet potatoes 135. Amasake doughnuts 45. Rice loaf 152. Apple butter 12. Bancha tea *Dinner* 1b. Pressure-cooked brown rice 69. Split pea macaroni soup 30. Nori nitsuke (leftover) 137. Cabbage, celery, daikon nuka pickles
18. Cabbage, onion, carrot miso soup 1b. Pressure-cooked brown rice 180. Daikon, daikon leaves, horsetail nitsuke 94. Muffins 69,178. Macaroni soup *mixed with* Sweet potato baked in ashes 137. Daikon nuka pickles	**Friday, April 20**	*Tea Time* 94. Muffins 45. Rice loaf 152. Apple butter *Dinner* 1b. Pressure-cooked brown rice 24,25. Kasha *with* Onion sesame sauce 55. Cabbage nitsuke 21a. Tossed salad 31. Apple pie
177. Bracken, onion, carrot miso soup 1b. Pressure-cooked brown rice 175. Broccoli and collard green nitsuke 137. Cabbage, celery, daikon nuka pickles *Mirimichi Camp ends after dinner.*	**Saturday, April 21**	1b. Pressure-cooked brown rice 2C. Mugwort mochi 2a. Mochi soup 2b. Azuki chestnut mochi (similar, see 27.) 2c. Walnut mochi 2d. Mochi with kinako 66. Swiss chard ohitashi with bonita flakes 14. Daikon nuka pickles
18. Swiss chard, onion, carrot miso soup 1b. Pressure-cooked brown rice 175. Vegetable nitsuke (leftover) 94. Azuki bean muffins 137. Cabbage, celery, daikon nuka pickles	**Sunday, April 22**	1b. Pressure-cooked brown rice 181. Deep-fried fish 128. Gyoza with lemon sauce (frozen) 114. Lettuce, saifun salad

Breakfast		*Dinner*
28. Wakame, onion, carrot miso soup 1b. Pressure-cooked brown rice 19. Collard green, celery nitsuke 99. Wheat cream 14. Daikon nuka pickles	**Monday, April 23**	1b. Pressure-cooked brown rice 50. Millet with chick pea sauce 21a. Tossed salad 14. Daikon nuka pickles
1b. Pressure-cooked brown rice 159. Koi-koku (frozen) 182. Dried zucchini, broccoli nitsuke 14. Daikon nuka pickles	**Tuesday, April 24**	*Cooking Class* 1b. Pressure-cooked brown rice 120. Tuna shish-kebab with barbecue sauce 176. Lentil soup 183. Cooked vegetable salad miso ai (lemon miso dressing)
176. Lentil soup (with miso added) 1b. Pressure-cooked brown rice 13. Natto with pickled daikon leaves 22c. Tempura crumbs (with leftover nitsuke) 15. Chinese cabbage nuka pickles	**Wednesday, April 25**	1b. Pressure-cooked brown rice 53. Clear soup with whole wheat spaghetti 91. Saifun nitsuke 14. Daikon nuka pickles
18. Daikon, daikon leaves, cauliflower leaves, carrot miso soup 1b. Pressure-cooked brown rice 55. Cabbage nitsuke 58. French bread 14. Daikon nuka pickles	**Thursday, April 26**	1b. Pressure-cooked brown rice 24,25. Kasha *with* Onion sesame sauce 133. Yam, carrot nitsuke 14. Daikon nuka pickles
18. Daikon, daikon leaves, cauliflower leaves, carrot miso soup 1b. Pressure-cooked brown rice 49. Rice cream 54. Broccoli nitsuke 14,15. Daikon, Chinese cabbage nuka pickles	**Friday, April 27**	80b. Home-made tofu, watercress miso soup (similar) 1b. Pressure-cooked brown rice 22a. Vegetable tempura 23. Grated daikon 184. Cabbage, red radish root and leaves pressed salad

Breakfast		*Dinner*
28. Wakame, tofu miso soup 1b. Pressure-cooked brown rice 100. Okara nitsuke 137. Cabbage, daikon nuka pickles	**Saturday, April 28**	1b. Pressure-cooked brown rice 264. Kasha croquettes with okara, mashed (similar) 37. Bechamel sauce with sweet potato 183. Cooked vegetable salad miso ai
28. Wakame miso soup 1b. Pressure-cooked brown rice 82,152. Waffles *with* Home-made apple butter 50. Chick pea sauce (leftover) 14. Daikon nuka pickles	**Sunday, April 29**	1b. Pressure-cooked brown rice 185. Omelette 91. Saifun nitsuke 184. Cabbage, red radish root and leaves pressed salad
28. Wakame miso soup 1b. Pressure-cooked brown rice 92. Mustard green nitsuke 99. Wheat cream 14,15. Daikon, Chinese cabbage nuka pickles	**Monday, April 30**	1b. Pressure-cooked brown rice 2C. Mugwort mochi 2d. Mochi with amasake and kinako 47. Cauliflower with kuzu sauce 72. Kombu, nori nitsuke 14,15. Daikon, cabbage nuka pickles

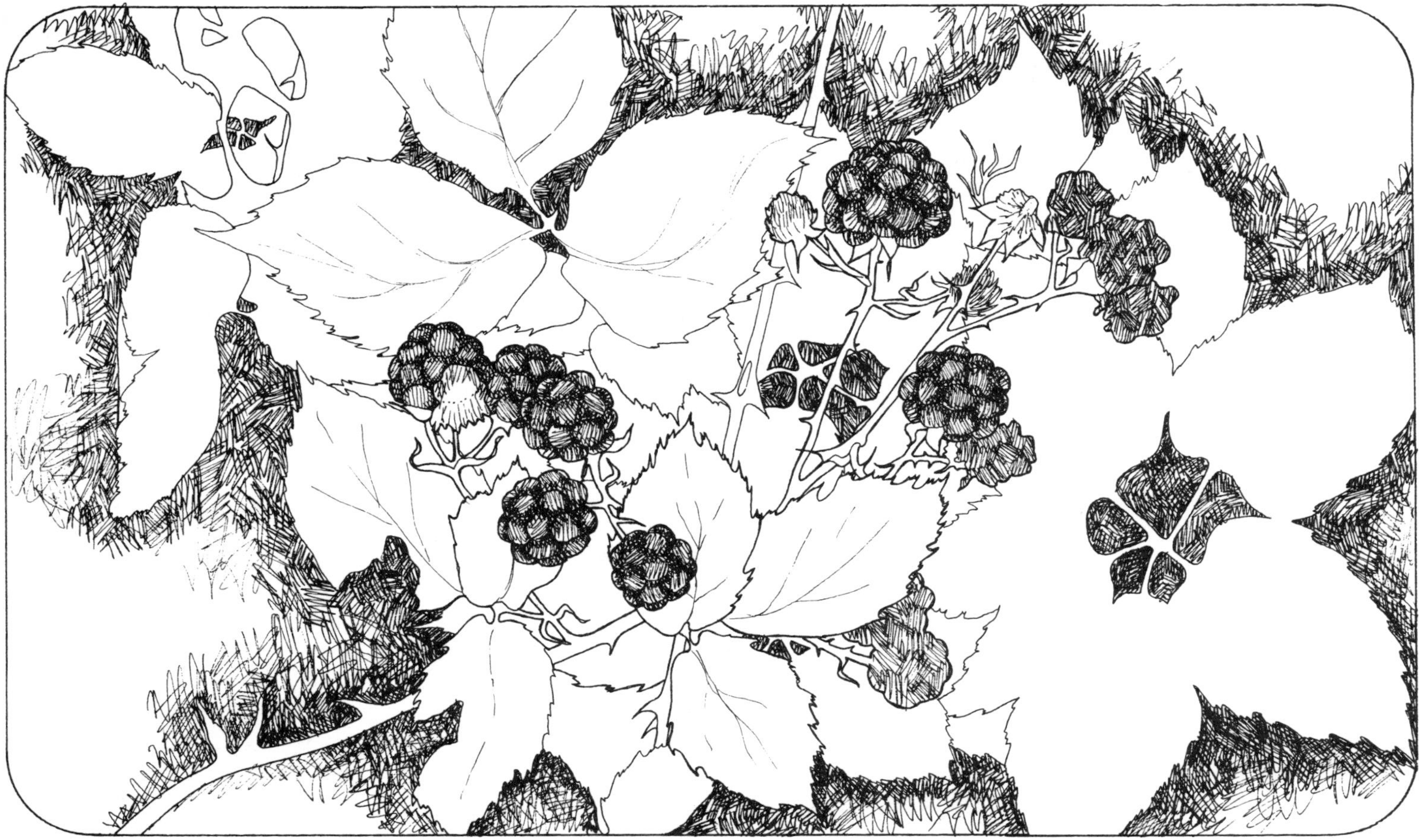

May

Breakfast		Dinner
18. Turnip, turnip top, onion, carrot miso soup 1a. Azuki bean rice 186. Hijiki nitsuke 14. Daikon nuka pickles	**Tuesday, May 1**	*Cooking Class* 1b. Pressure-cooked brown rice 187. Vegetables with curry sauce 188. Mekabu nitsuke 189. Corn bread 190. Apple, chestnut ring 14. Daikon nuka pickles
18. Turnip, turnip leaves, onion, carrot miso soup 1b. Pressure-cooked brown rice 100. Okara (leftover) 186,72 Hijiki (leftover) *mixed with* Nori nitsuke (leftover) 137. Cabbage nuka pickles	**Wednesday, May 2**	1b. Pressure-cooked brown rice 24,25. Kasha *with* Sesame onion sauce 91,22c. Saifun nitsuke *with* Tempura crumbs 137. Daikon, cabbage nuka pickles
18. Turnip, turnip leaves, onion, carrot miso soup with pan-fried tofu 1b. Pressure-cooked brown rice 19. Cabbage and collard green nitsuke 137. Cabbage, daikon nuka pickles	**Thursday, May 3**	1b. Pressure-cooked brown rice 29. Pan-fried spaghetti 21a. Tossed salad 187. Vegetables with curry sauce 137. Cabbage nuka pickles
18. Leek, cauliflower leaves, cabbage, carrot miso soup 1b. Pressure-cooked brown rice 19. Vegetable nitsuke (leftover) 14. Daikon nuka pickles	**Friday, May 4**	*Boys' Day Eve* 1b. Pressure-cooked brown rice 2C. Mugwort mochi 2a. Mochi soup 2b. Azuki chestnut mochi (see 27.) 2c. Walnut mochi 2d. Kinako mochi 66. Swiss chard ohitashi with bonita flakes 15. Chinese cabbage nuka pickles
18. Leek, cauliflower leaves, cabbage, carrot miso soup 1b. Pressure-cooked brown rice 92. Mustard green, cabbage nitsuke 13. Natto with pickled daikon leaves 14,15. Daikon, cabbage nuka pickles	**Saturday, May 5**	162. Seitan goma rice 191. Spaghetti with tomato sauce 21a. Tossed salad

Breakfast		*Dinner*
Breakfast out. *(Gone fishing)*	**Sunday, May 6**	1b. Pressure-cooked brown rice Salmon, canned at home 23. Grated daikon 29. Fried spaghetti (leftover) 66. Mustard green ohitashi 14,15. Daikon, cabbage nuka pickles
18. Leek, cabbage, carrot miso soup 1b. Pressure-cooked brown rice 19. Collard green, mustard green nitsuke 2C. Mugwort mochi (leftover) 2b,c,d. Mochi (leftover) 14,15. Daikon, cabbage nuka pickles	**Monday, May 7**	1b. Pressure-cooked brown rice 164. Noodle croquettes with kasha 37. Bechamel sauce 66 Swiss chard ohitashi with kirigoma 14. Daikon nuka pickles
18,2C. Leek miso soup *with* Mugwort mochi 1b. Pressure-cooked brown rice 49. Rice cream 97. Scallion miso 54. Broccoli nitsuke 14. Daikon nuka pickles	**Tuesday, May 8**	*Cooking Class* 1b. Pressure-cooked brown rice 192. Metropolitan soup 151. Stuffed cabbage with white sauce 14. Daikon, daikon leaves nuka pickles 193. Tahini custard
18. Leek, cabbage, carrot miso soup 1b. Pressure-cooked brown rice 13. Natto with pickled daikon leaves 19. Vegetable nitsuke (leftover) 14,15. Daikon, cabbage nuka pickles	**Wednesday, May 9**	1b. Pressure-cooked brown rice 47. Cauliflower with kuzu sauce 72. Kombu, mekabu, nori nitsuke (similar) 15. Cabbage nuka pickles
52,2C. Vegetable ojiya *with* Mugwort mochi 1b. Pressure-cooked brown rice 49. Rice cream 55. Cabbage nitsuke 14,15. Daikon, cabbage nuka pickles	**Thursday, May 10**	1b. Pressure-cooked brown rice 38,37. Kasha croquettes (leftover) *with* Bechamel sauce 66. Swiss chard, outer lettuce leaves ohitashi with bonita flakes 21a. Tossed salad 194. Amasake cookies

Breakfast		Dinner
18,2C. Cauliflower leaves, onion, cabbage, carrot miso soup *with* Mugwort mochi 1b. Pressure-cooked brown rice 100. Okara nitsuke 14,15. Daikon, cabbage nuka pickles	**Friday, May 11**	1b. Pressure-cooked brown rice 50. Millet with chick pea sauce 30. Nori nitsuke 14. Daikon nuka pickles 194. Amasake cookies
18. Cauliflower leaves, onion, cabbage, carrot miso soup 1b. Pressure-cooked brown rice 55,22c. Cabbage nitsuke *with* Tempura crumbs 14,15. Daikon, cabbage nuka pickles	**Saturday, May 12**	1b. Pressure-cooked brown rice 120. Fresh tuna shish-kebab 50. Chick pea sauce (leftover) 194. Amasake cookies 15. Chinese cabbage nuka pickles
Picnic 146. Norimake sushi 195. Fresh green pea rice 147. Piroshki 14. Daikon nuka pickles 194. Amasake cookies	**Sunday, May 13**	18. Vegetable miso soup 1b. Pressure-cooked brown rice 146. Norimake sushi (leftover) 14. Daikon nuka pickles
28. Wakame, onion, cabbage, carrot miso soup 1b. Pressure-cooked brown rice 146. Norimake sushi (leftover) 50. Chick pea sauce with green vegetable 14. Daikon nuka pickles	**Monday, May 14**	1b. Pressure-cooked brown rice 38,47. Kasha croquettes (leftover) *with* Cauliflower with kuzu sauce and barbecue sauce 39. Lettuce goma ai 14,15. Daikon, cabbage nuka pickles
18,2C. Daikon, daikon leaves, onion, carrot miso soup *with* Mugwort mochi 1b. Pressure-cooked brown rice 99. Wheat cream 100. Okara nitsuke (leftover) 14,15. Daikon, cabbage nuka pickles	**Tuesday, May 15**	*Cooking Class* 197. Onion cream miso soup 1b. Pressure-cooked brown rice 196. Chirashi sushi 48. Parsnip, celery nitsuke 185. Cabbage, daikon top and scallion pressed salad (similar) 194. Amasake cookies

Breakfast		*Dinner*
1a. Azuki bean rice 197. Onion cream miso soup 54. Broccoli nitsuke 14,15. Daikon, cabbage nuka pickles	**Wednesday, May 16**	1b. Pressure-cooked brown rice 186. Hijiki nitsuke 56. Garlic French bread 80. Fresh home-made tofu with bonita flakes, sliced scallions and grated ginger 14,15. Daikon, cabbage nuka pickles
18,2C. Daikon, onion, carrot miso soup *with* Mugwort mochi 1b. Pressure-cooked brown rice 99. Wheat cream 55. Cabbage nitsuke with sesame butter 100. Okara nitsuke	**Thursday, May 17**	1b. Pressure-cooked brown rice 65,37. Millet croquettes *with* Bechamel sauce 21a,76a. Tossed salad with crab meat *and* Mayonnaise dressing
18. Daikon, onion, carrot miso soup 1b. Pressure-cooked brown rice 92. Mustard green nitsuke 14,15. Daikon, cabbage nuka pickles	**Friday, May 18**	1b. Pressure-cooked brown rice 22a,53. Vegetable tempura udon *with* Broth 140. Dried daikon nitsuke 141. Condiment pickles 185. Cabbage, carrot, scallion pressed salad (similar)
18. Miso soup (leftover) 1b. Pressure-cooked brown rice 32. Kidney beans with miso 14. Daikon leaves nuka pickles	**Saturday, May 19**	*Gone to Chico.*
Gone to Chico.	**Sunday, May 20**	28. Wakame, onion, carrot miso soup 1b. Pressure-cooked brown rice Salmon, canned at home 23. Grated daikon and ginger with tamari 32. Kidney beans with miso (leftover) 14. Daikon nuka pickles

Breakfast		*Dinner*
28. Wakame, onion, carrot, cabbage miso soup 1b. Pressure-cooked brown rice 63. Collard green nitsuke 14. Daikon nuka pickles	**Monday, May 21**	*Dinner for Michio Kushi* 1b. Pressure-cooked brown rice 2a. Mochi soup 2d. Kinako mochi with amasake 198. Cooked shad with fresh grated daikon 91. Saifun nitsuke 66. Shingiku, swiss chard ohitashi 14. Daikon, daikon leaves nuka pickles
18. Cabbage, onion, carrot miso soup 1b. Pressure-cooked brown rice 63. Vegetable nitsuke (leftover) 14. Daikon and daikon leaves nuka pickles	**Tuesday, May 22**	*Cooking Class* 1b. Pressure-cooked brown rice 29. Pan-fried whole wheat spaghetti 199. Soybean soup 21a. Tossed salad 315. Orange kanten (similar)
18,199. Miso soup (leftover) *mixed with* Soybean soup (leftover) 1b. Pressure-cooked brown rice 55. Cabbage nitsuke 14. Daikon nuka pickles	**Wednesday, May 23**	1b. Pressure-cooked brown rice 30. Nori nitsuke 91. Saifun nitsuke (leftover) 14. Daikon, daikon leaves nuka pickles
177. Buckwheat dumpling miso soup 1b. Pressure-cooked brown rice 54. Broccoli nitsuke 14. Daikon nuka pickles	**Thursday, May 24**	1b. Pressure-cooked brown rice 29. Fried spaghetti (leftover) 200. Ohsawa corn bread 21a. Tossed salad
18. Cabbage, onion, carrot miso soup 1b. Pressure-cooked brown rice 19. Collard green, onion, carrot nitsuke 14,15. Daikon, cabbage nuka pickles	**Friday, May 25**	1b. Pressure-cooked brown rice 176. Lentil soup 128. Pan-fried gyoza 201. Boiled carrots 14. Daikon nuka pickles 31. Apple pie

Breakfast		Dinner
176. Lentil soup with miso 1b. Pressure-cooked brown rice 83,152. Waffles *with* Home-made apple butter 13. Natto with pickled daikon leaves 15. Chinese cabbage nuka pickles	**Saturday, May 26**	119. Fried rice 133. Carrot, yam nitsuke 14. Daikon nuka pickles 31. Apple pie
Gone to Chico.	**Sunday, May 27**	*Gone to Chico.*
18. Collard green, onion, carrot miso soup 202. Bamboo shoot rice 54. Broccoli nitsuke 14,15. Daikon, cabbage nuka pickles	**Monday, May 28**	1b. Pressure-cooked brown rice 47. Cauliflower with kuzu sauce 30. Nori nitsuke 15. Chinese cabbage nuka pickles
18. Collard green, onion, carrot miso soup 1b. Pressure-cooked brown rice 55. Cabbage nitsuke 14,15. Daikon, cabbage nuka pickles	**Tuesday, May 29**	*Cooking Class* 1b. Pressure-cooked brown rice 22a. Vegetable tempura 53. Clear soup with udon noodles 140. Dried daikon nitsuke 23. Grated daikon, sliced scallion (condiment for udon) 16a. Momi nori (condiment for udon) 203. Strawberry, white raisin kanten 15. Chinese cabbage nuka pickles
18. Cabbage, onion, carrot miso soup 1b. Pressure-cooked brown rice 54,55. Vegetable nitsuke (leftover) 13. Natto with pickled daikon leaves	**Wednesday, May 30**	1b. Pressure-cooked brown rice 10. Baked fresh shad 23. Grated ginger, daikon 17. Chick pea sauce 87a. Seitan 335. Gluten starch pudding
18. Cabbage, onion, carrot miso soup 1b. Pressure-cooked brown rice 140,22c. Dried daikon nitsuke *with* Tempura crumbs 58. French bread 14,15. Daikon, cabbage nuka pickles	**Thursday, May 31**	*GOMF Director's Meeting* 1b. Pressure-cooked brown rice 87e. Gluten cutlet vegetable kebabs 80a. Tofu shingiku clear soup 114. Saifun salad 203. Strawberry, white raisin kanten 14. Daikon nuka pickles

June

Breakfast		Dinner
1a. Azuki bean rice 28. Wakame, onion, cabbage miso soup 54. Broccoli nitsuke 137. Cabbage nuka pickles	**Friday, June 1**	1b. Pressure-cooked brown rice 69. Split pea macaroni soup 151. Stuffed cabbage with white sauce 30. Nori nitsuke 58. Home-made French bread 137. Cabbage nuka pickles
Gone to Chico.	**Saturday, June 2**	*Gone to Chico.*
28. Wakame, onion, cabbage miso soup 1b. Pressure-cooked brown rice 13. Natto with pickled daikon leaves 137. Cabbage nuka pickles	**Sunday, June 3**	1b. Pressure-cooked brown rice 121. White rice 10. Baked shad with grated ginger, tamari 137. Cabbage nuka pickles
28. Wakame, onion, carrot miso soup 1b. Pressure-cooked brown rice 35. Onion miso 57. Carrot, sesame seed nitsuke 137. Cabbage nuka pickles	**Monday, June 4**	1b. Pressure-cooked brown rice 53,22c. Udon with clear broth *with* Tempura crumbs 75. Northern white beans with white rice miso 137. Cabbage nuka pickles
18,2C. Miso soup with watercress *with* Mugwort mochi 1b. Pressure-cooked brown rice 55. Cabbage nitsuke 137. Daikon, cabbage nuka pickles	**Tuesday, June 5**	1b. Pressure-cooked brown rice 47,87d. Broccoli with kuzu sauce (similar) *with* Gluten cutlets 21a. Tossed salad 135. Amasake doughnuts

Breakfast		Dinner
18. Turnip, turnip top, onion, carrot miso soup 1b. Pressure-cooked brown rice 55. Cabbage nitsuke (leftover) 13. Natto with pickled daikon leaves 137. Daikon, cabbage nuka pickles	**Wednesday, June 6**	*Mirimichi Camp begins* 1b. Pressure-cooked brown rice 204. Sauteed purple cabbage, onion, carrot, green pepper 58. French bread 10,37. Baked shad with grated ginger *and* Bechamel sauce 135. Amasake doughnuts Fresh cherries
28. Wakame, onion, turnip, turnip green, carrot miso soup 1b. Pressure-cooked brown rice 136. Oatmeal 54. Broccoli nitsuke	**Thursday, June 7**	1b. Pressure-cooked brown rice 112. Fried striped bass with kuzu sauce 21a. Tossed salad 137. Watermelon rind nuka pickles 205. Cherry pie
18. Beet, onion, carrot miso soup 1b. Pressure-cooked brown rice 49. Rice cream 92. Mustard green nitsuke 137. Daikon, watermelon rind nuka pickles	**Friday, June 8**	1b. Pressure-cooked brown rice 235. Somen with clear broth 92. Mustard green nitsuke (leftover) 137. Chinese cabbage, watermelon rind nuka pickles
18,53. Fresh chicory miso soup *mixed with* Clear soup with udon 96. Rice kayu 136. Oatmeal 46. Onion, carrot with oily miso 137. Daikon, cabbage nuka pickles	**Saturday, June 9**	206. Barley - brown rice 207. Salmon head with curry sauce 140. Dried daikon nitsuke 201. Boiled yams (similar) 137. Cabbage nuka pickles
18. Daikon, daikon leaves, carrot, shiitake mushroom miso soup 1b. Pressure-cooked brown rice 208. Corn meal 55. Cabbage, nitsuke 137. Daikon, cabbage nuka pickles	**Sunday, June 10**	1b. Pressure-cooked brown rice 209,17. Bulghur *with* Chick pea sauce 30. Nori nitsuke 137. Cabbage nuka pickles

Breakfast		*Dinner*
18. Cabbage, onion, carrot miso soup 1b. Pressure-cooked brown rice 49. Rice cream 92. Mustard green nitsuke 137. Daikon, cabbage nuka pickles	**Monday, June 11**	1b. Pressure-cooked brown rice 210,37. Bulghur croquettes *with* Bechamel sauce 21a. Tossed salad 17,140. Chick pea sauce (leftover) *with* Dried daikon nitsuke (leftover) 211. Fresh cherry, apple juice kanten
28. Wakame, onion, cabbage miso soup 1b. Pressure-cooked brown rice 208. Corn meal 212. Creamed cabbage 137. Cabbage, daikon nuka pickles	**Tuesday, June 12**	1b. Pressure-cooked brown rice 22a. Vegetable tempura 23. Grated ginger and daikon 137. Chinese cabbage nuka pickles
28. Wakame, daikon, onion miso soup 1b. Pressure-cooked brown rice 213. Collard green, broccoli, sweet potato nitsuke 137. Daikon, cabbage nuka pickles	**Wednesday, June 13**	214. Rice salad 47,53. Udon *with* Kuzu sauce 163. Sauteed onion, potato, green pepper 137. Cabbage nuka pickles
52. Daikon, turnip, onion ojiya with mochi 136. Oatmeal 92. Bok choy, onion nitsuke (similar) 137. Daikon, daikon leaves nuka pickles	**Thursday, June 14**	1b. Pressure-cooked brown rice 24,25. Kasha *with* Sesame onion sauce 75. Northern white beans with white rice miso 14. Dried daikon nuka pickles 215a. Raisin buns with strawberry topping
18. Daikon, turnip, carrot miso soup 1a. Azuki bean rice 49. Rice cream 54. Broccoli, onion nitsuke 137. Daikon, cabbage nuka pickles	**Friday, June 15**	1b. Pressure-cooked brown rice 87d. Gluten cutlets 21a. Tossed salad 23. Grated daikon, carrot 24,25. Kasha (leftover) *mixed with* Northern white beans (leftover) with chickweed 174. Raisin roll

Breakfast		Dinner
18. Daikon, daikon leaves, onion, carrot miso soup 1b. Pressure-cooked brown rice 208. Corn meal 46. Onion, carrot with oily miso 137. Cucumber, cabbage nuka pickles	**Saturday, June 16**	1b. Pressure-cooked brown rice 29. Pan-fried spaghetti 61. Green pea nitsuke 137. Daikon nuka pickles
177. Beet, beet top, onion, carrot miso soup with buckwheat dumplings 1b. Pressure-cooked brown rice 216. Onion, zucchini nitsuke 137. Chinese cabbage nuka pickles	**Sunday, June 17**	177. Miso soup (leftover) 1b. Pressure-cooked brown rice 47. Snow peas with kuzu sauce (similar) 30. Nori nitsuke 205. Cherry pie
18. Daikon, daikon leaves, onion, carrot miso soup 1b. Pressure-cooked brown rice 55. Cabbage nitsuke 30. Nori nitsuke (leftover) 94,61. Muffins *with* Green pea filling 137. Cucumber, watermelon rind nuka pickles	**Monday, June 18**	*Ocean Camp begins* 1b. Pressure-cooked brown rice 24. Kasha 213. Sweet potato, carrot, bok choy nitsuke (similar) 137. Celery, cabbage nuka pickles
28. Fresh seaweed, onion, carrot miso soup 1b. Pressure-cooked brown rice 136. Oatmeal 216. Zucchini nitsuke 137. Celery, cucumber nuka pickles	**Tuesday, June 19**	1b. Pressure-cooked brown rice 181. Deep-fried trout 69. Split pea and macaroni soup 91. Saifun nitsuke 217. Cucumber salad
69. Macaroni soup (leftover) with miso 1b. Pressure-cooked brown rice 91. Saifun nitsuke 218. Cold salmon with gravy 137. Daikon nuka pickles *Ocean Camp ends*	**Wednesday, June 20**	*Back home* 1b. Pressure-cooked brown rice 219. Sauteed onion, potato with salmon, egg 80. Tofu with grated ginger condiment 184. Cucumber, cabbage pressed salad

Breakfast	Day	Dinner
28. Wakame, onion, celery, carrot miso soup 1b. Pressure-cooked brown rice 32. Pinto bean with miso (similar) 175. Bok choy, broccoli nitsuke 137. Daikon, Chinese cabbage nuka pickles	**Thursday, June 21**	*Mirimichi Camp continues* 1b. Pressure-cooked brown rice 140. Dried daikon nitsuke 168. Baked yams (similar) 21a. Tossed green salad
18. Turnip, onion, carrot miso soup 1b. Pressure-cooked brown rice 136. Oatmeal 19. Collard green, onion nitsuke	**Friday, June 22**	1b. Pressure-cooked brown rice 209,47. Bulghur *with* Snow pea kuzu sauce 72. Nori, kombu nitsuke 21a. Tossed salad 137. Cabbage, daikon nuka pickles 215. Raisin buns
177. Turnip, endive, onion miso soup with buckwheat dumpling 1b. Pressure-cooked brown rice 208. Corn meal 175. Broccoli, zucchini nitsuke (similar) 184. Cucumber, cabbage pressed salad	**Saturday, June 23**	1b. Pressure-cooked brown rice 192. Metropolitan soup 128. Baked gyoza with lemon sauce 137. Cucumber, cabbage nuka pickles 205. Cherry pie
28. Fresh seaweed, onion, carrot miso soup 1a. Azuki bean rice 94,128. Vegetable pancakes (batter similar, *mixed with* Gyoza stuffing) 137. Daikon, cabbage nuka pickles	**Sunday, June 24**	220. Tofu, snow pea white rice miso soup 1b. Pressure-cooked brown rice 2C,b,c,d. Mochi with coverings 140. Dried daikon nitsuke 137. Cucumber nuka pickles
18. Turnip, onion, carrot miso soup 1b. Pressure-cooked brown rice 216. Zucchini nitsuke 137. Daikon, cucumber nuka pickles	**Monday, June 25**	1b. Pressure-cooked brown rice 222,47. Somen *with* Kuzu sauce 221. Hijiki, carrot nitsuke 90. Oatmeal cookies 27. Azuki raisin kanten (similar) 137. Cucumber nuka pickles

Breakfast		Dinner
18,222. Cabbage, onion, carrot miso soup *with* Somen (leftover) 1b. Pressure-cooked brown rice 100. Okara nitsuke 137. Cucumber, cabbage nuka pickles	**Tuesday, June 26**	1b. Pressure-cooked brown rice 147. Piroshki 80a. Tofu, snow pea clear soup 21a. Tossed salad 211. Mixed dried fruit kanten (raisin and apricot) with fresh cherries
18. Turnip, onion, carrot miso soup 1b. Pressure-cooked brown rice 216. Zucchini onion nitsuke 137. Celery, cucumber nuka pickles	**Wednesday, June 27**	214. Rice salad 147. Piroshki (leftover) with kuzu sauce 91. Saifun nitsuke 72. Nori, kombu nitsuke 223. Sesame balls Watermelon
18. Cabbage, onion, carrot miso soup 32. Kidney beans with miso 91. Saifun nitsuke (leftover) 214. Rice salad (leftover) 137. Cucumber, watermelon rind nuka pickles	**Thursday, June 28**	*Mirimichi Summer Camp ends.* *Dinner Out.*
Gone to Chico.	**Friday, June 29**	*Gone to Chico.*
1b. Pressure-cooked brown rice 47. Burdock, carrot, string bean with kuzu sauce (similar) 186. Hijiki nitsuke 224. Wakame cucumber salad	**Saturday, June 30**	1b. Pressure-cooked brown rice 235. Somen with clear broth 186. Hijiki nitsuke 137. Cabbage nuka pickles 225. French bread pudding

July

Breakfast		Dinner
28. Wakame, onion, carrot miso soup 1a. Azuki bean rice 216,55. Zucchini, cabbage nitsuke 137. Cucumber, daikon nuka pickles	**Sunday, July 1**	1b. Pressure-cooked brown rice 22a. Vegetable tempura 23. Grated daikon and carrot 137. Chinese cabbage nuka pickles
28. Wakame miso soup with tofu 1b. Pressure-cooked brown rice 136. Oatmeal 17. Chick pea sauce (with sweet potato nitsuke) 137. Cucumber nuka pickles	**Monday, July 2**	1b. Pressure-cooked brown rice 120. Fresh tuna shish-kebab 140. Dried daikon nitsuke 21a. Tossed green salad
18. Cabbage, beet, onion miso soup 1b. Pressure-cooked brown rice 216. Zucchini nitsuke 137. Cucumber, watermelon rind nuka pickles	**Tuesday, July 3**	1b. Pressure-cooked brown rice 22a,53. Tempura udon with clear broth (leftover) 140. Dried daikon nitsuke (leftover) 137. Cucumber, cabbage nuka pickles
18. Miso soup (leftover) with tofu 1b. Pressure-cooked brown rice 17. Chick pea sauce (leftover) 13. Natto with pickled daikon leaves 137. Cucumber nuka pickles	**Wednesday, July 4**	*July 4th Ceremony* 1b. Pressure-cooked brown rice 226a. Tomato - cheese pizza 80. Cold tofu with bonita flakes condiment 92. Takana nitsuke (similar) 137. Cucumber nuka pickles
18. Cabbage, onion, carrot, scallion, nori miso soup 1b. Pressure-cooked brown rice 227b. String bean, zucchini nitsuke 137. Cucumber, watermelon rind nuka pickles	**Thursday, July 5**	*Tea Time* 58. French bread 228. Apple butter made from dried apples *Dinner* 1b. Pressure-cooked brown rice 29. Pan-fried spaghetti 72. Nori kombu nitsuke 137. Cucumber, watermelon rind nuka pickles

July 6 through August 16

Away on lecture tour.

Suggested recipes for summer: 229 - 239.

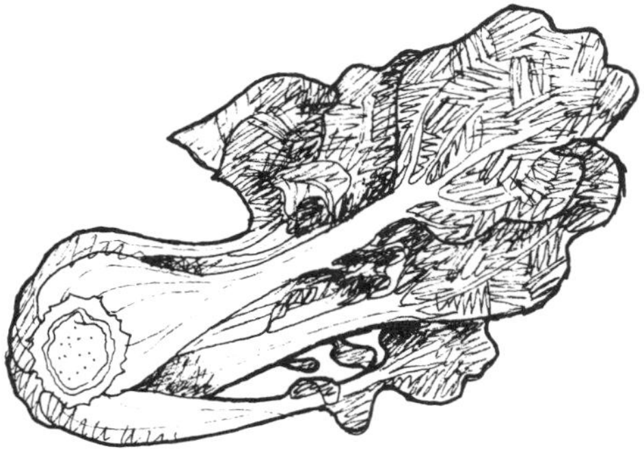

August

Breakfast		Dinner
French Meadows Camp begins 28. Wakame, onion, cabbage miso soup 1b. Pressure-cooked brown rice 236. Baked rice balls with tamari 137. Cucumber nuka pickles	**Friday, August 17**	1a. Azuki bean rice 240. Summer vegetable macaroni soup 241b. Corn on the cob, outdoor cooking 216. Crookneck squash, onion nitsuke 15. Chinese cabbage nuka pickles
177. Vegetable miso soup with buckwheat dumplings 1b. Pressure-cooked brown rice 92. Mustard green, onion nitsuke 221. Hijiki, carrot nitsuke 137. Cucumber, daikon leaves nuka pickles	**Saturday, August 18**	1b. Pressure-cooked brown rice 47. Vegetables with kuzu sauce 30. Nori nitsuke 21a,b. Tossed salad with French dressing
18. Turnip, onion, carrot miso soup 1b. Pressure-cooked brown rice 91. Saifun nitsuke 242,243. Top of stove bread *with* Pear butter 137. Cucumber nuka pickles	**Sunday, August 19**	1b. Pressure-cooked brown rice 176. Lentil soup 29. Pan-fried whole wheat spaghetti 26. Boiled beets 15. Chinese cabbage nuka pickles
28. Wakame, onion, cabbage miso soup 1b. Pressure-cooked brown rice 49. Rice cream 216. Summer squash nitsuke Watermelon	**Monday, August 20**	1b. Pressure-cooked brown rice 69. Split pea macaroni soup 35. Onion miso 137. Cucumber, cabbage nuka pickles
244. Barley miso soup 1b. Pressure-cooked brown rice 245. Tekka miso 227a. String bean, celery nitsuke with sesame butter 137. Watermelon rind nuka pickles	**Tuesday, August 21**	1b. Pressure-cooked brown rice 246,160. Polenta potage *with* Whole wheat noodle salad with sesame butter dressing 140. Dried daikon nitsuke 137. Cabbage, celery nuka pickles

Breakfast		Dinner
18. Cabbage, onion, carrot miso soup 1b. Pressure-cooked brown rice 34,246. Butternut squash, onion nitsuke *with* Polenta potage (leftover) 140. Dried daikon nitsuke (leftover) 137. Celery, cabbage nuka pickles Watermelon	**Wednesday, August 22**	134. Gomoku rice 115. Egg drop soup 114. Saifun salad with mayonnaise dressing
18. Onion, turnip, carrot miso soup 1b. Pressure-cooked brown rice 133. Sweet potato, carrot nitsuke 72. Nori, kombu nitsuke 15. Chinese cabbage nuka pickles	**Thursday, August 23**	1b. Pressure-cooked brown rice 187. Vegetables with curry sauce 97. Scallion miso 15. Chinese cabbage nuka pickles
18. Onion, cabbage, crookneck squash miso soup 1b. Pressure-cooked brown rice 26. Boiled beets with tops 227a. String bean nitsuke with sesame butter 137. Cucumber nuka pickles Watermelon	**Friday, August 24**	1b. Pressure-cooked brown rice 16. Buckwheat noodles with clear soup 221. Hijiki, onion nitsuke (similar) 21a. Tossed salad
177. Buckwheat dumpling miso soup 1b. Pressure-cooked brown rice 216. Zucchini onion nitsuke 137. Watermelon rind nuka pickles	**Saturday, August 25**	1a. Azuki bean rice 248. Clear soup with cucumber 22a. Vegetable tempura 23. Grated daikon and carrot 66. Ohitashi 249. Apple - pear kanten
18. Butternut squash, onion miso soup 1b. Pressure-cooked brown rice 22a. Vegetable tempura (leftover) 212. Creamed cabbage 137. Watermelon rind nuka pickles	**Sunday, August 26**	*French Meadows Camp ends.* *On the Road.*

Breakfast			Dinner
18. Onion, turnip, carrot miso soup 1b. Pressure-cooked brown rice 136. Oatmeal 55. Cabbage nitsuke 15. Chinese cabbage nuka pickles	**Monday, August 27**		1b. Pressure-cooked brown rice 17. Chick pea sauce 30. Nori nitsuke 137. Cabbage nuka pickles
18. Daikon, onion, carrot miso soup 1b. Pressure-cooked brown rice 227b. String bean, onion, carrot nitsuke 137. Cabbage, turnip nuka pickles	**Tuesday, August 28**		1b. Pressure-cooked brown rice 187. Vegetables with curry sauce 97. Scallion miso 137. Cucumber nuka pickles
18. Onion, carrot, Chinese cabbage miso soup 1b. Pressure-cooked brown rice 49. Rice cream 221. Hijiki - carrot nitsuke 137. Watermelon rind nuka pickles	**Wednesday, August 29**		41. Baked brown rice 250. Azuki with home-made whole wheat noodles 21a. Tossed salad 225. French bread pudding
18. Daikon, daikon leaves miso soup 1b. Pressure-cooked brown rice 32. Kidney beans with miso 13. Natto with pickled daikon leaves 137. Cabbage, turnip nuka pickles	**Thursday, August 30**		1b. Pressure-cooked brown rice 80a. Clear broth with tofu and shingiku 29. Pan-fried whole wheat spaghetti 251. Fried eggplant with lemon miso sauce 137. Chinese cabbage nuka pickles
28. Wakame, onion, cabbage, carrot miso soup 1b. Pressure-cooked brown rice 227b. String bean, zucchini, carrot nitsuke 137. Cabbage, cucumber nuka pickles	**Friday, August 31**		1b. Pressure-cooked brown rice 47. Cauliflower with kuzu sauce 72. Kombu, nori nitsuke 137. Cabbage, turnip nuka pickles

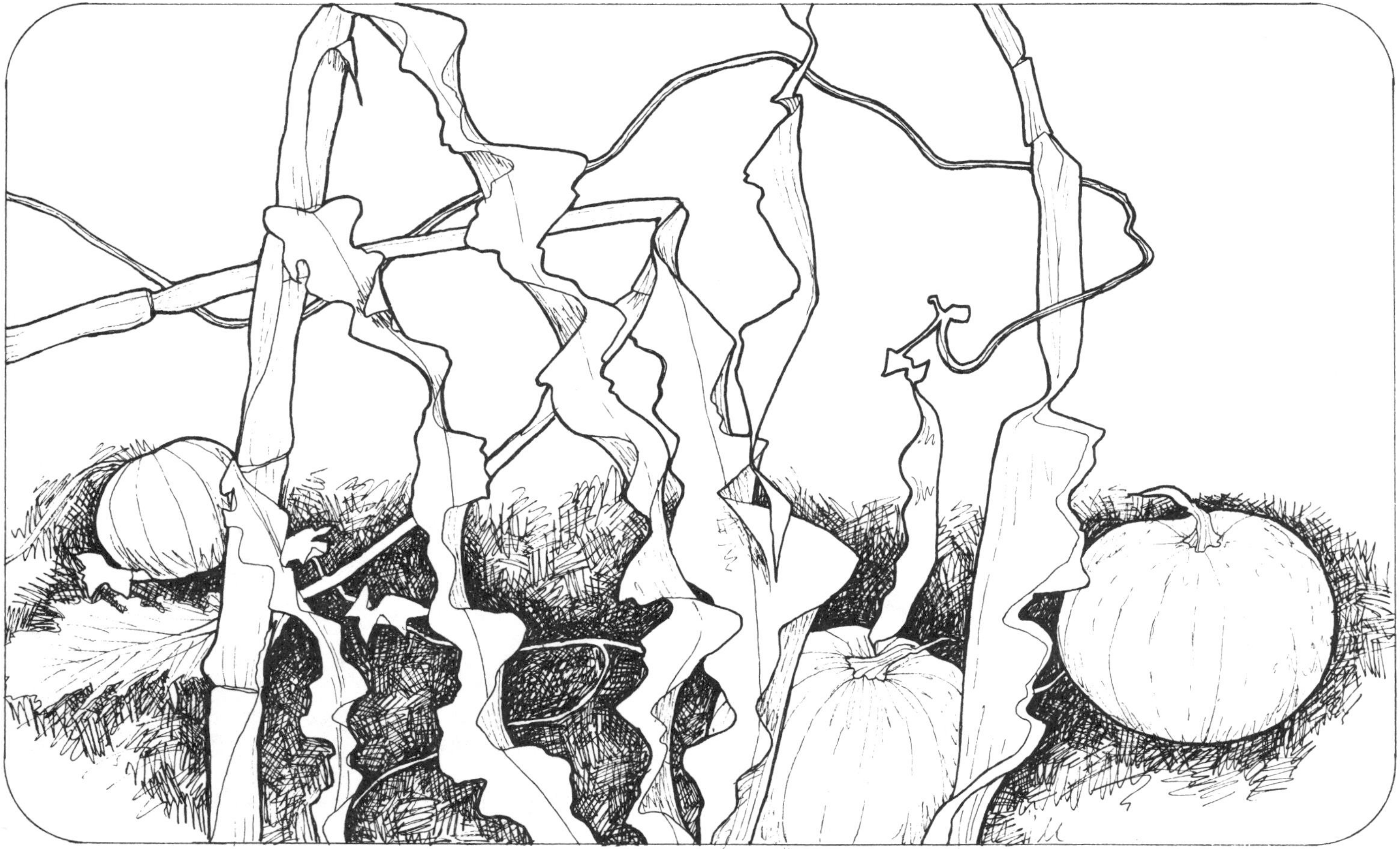

September

Breakfast				Dinner
28.	Wakame, onion, cabbage, carrot miso soup	**Saturday, September 1**	1b.	Pressure-cooked brown rice
1a.	Azuki bean rice		252,37.	Noodle gratin *with* Bechamel sauce
140.	Dried daikon nitsuke		241a.	Boiled corn on the cob
137.	Cabbage, turnip, eggplant nuka pickles		137.	Cabbage nuka pickles
28.	Wakame miso soup with tofu, watercress	**Sunday, September 2**	1b.	Pressure-cooked brown rice
1b.	Pressure-cooked brown rice		53,22c.	Clear soup with noodles *with* Tempura crumbs
19.	Collard green, onion nitsuke		16a,b.	Momi nori, sarashinegi
137.	Cucumber, cabbage nuka pickles		19.	Collard green nitsuke (leftover) with cooked corn
18.	String bean, onion, carrot miso soup	**Monday, September 3**	1b.	Pressure-cooked brown rice
1b.	Pressure-cooked brown rice		253.	Togan with kuzu sauce
216.	Zucchini - onion nitsuke		186.	Hijiki nitsuke
137.	Cucumber, cabbage nuka pickles		137.	Cucumber nuka pickles
18.	String bean, onion, carrot miso soup	**Tuesday, September 4**		*Tea Time for Labor Day*
1b.	Pressure-cooked brown rice		226a.	Tomato - cheese pizza
254.	Carrot, carrot top, fresh corn nitsuke		226a.	Tomato - salmon pizza
13.	Natto with pickled daikon leaves		226b.	Fresh vegetable pizza
137.	Cucumber, cabbage nuka pickles			*Dinner*
			1b.	Pressure-cooked brown rice
			24,25.	Kasha *with* Sesame sauce
			255.	Banana squash, string bean, onion nitsuke
			137.	Celery, cucumber nuka pickles
18.	Yellow crookneck squash, onion miso soup	**Wednesday, September 5**	1b.	Pressure-cooked brown rice
1b.	Pressure-cooked brown rice		91.	Saifun nitsuke
49.	Rice cream		257.	Green pepper with sauteed miso
256.	Cabbage, bean sprout, carrot nitsuke		137.	Cucumber, celery nuka pickles
137.	Cucumber, celery nuka pickles			

Breakfast		Dinner
18. Miso soup (leftover) with shingiku 1b. Pressure-cooked brown rice 258. Sweet potato, carrot, banana squash nitsuke 137. Cucumber, celery nuka pickles	**Thursday, September 6**	1b. Pressure-cooked brown rice 259. Tofu with mustard sauce 251. Fried eggplant with lemon miso sauce 137. Cabbage nuka pickles
18. Turnip, onion, carrot miso soup 1b. Pressure-cooked brown rice 19. Collard green, onion, carrot nitsuke 13. Natto with pickled daikon leaves 137. Cabbage nuka pickles	**Friday, September 7**	1b. Pressure-cooked brown rice 80a. Clear soup with tofu and shingiku 218. Cold salmon with gravy 66. Ohitashi 21a,b. Tossed salad with French dressing 157. Eggplant mustard pickles 174. Raisin roll
18. Bok choy, onion, carrot miso soup 1b. Pressure-cooked brown rice 208. Corn meal 186. Hijiki nitsuke (leftover) 91. Saifun nitsuke (leftover) 137. Cabbage nuka pickles	**Saturday, September 8**	1b. Pressure-cooked brown rice 38. Kasha croquettes 66. Shingiku ohitashi 21a. Tossed salad 137. Cucumber nuka pickles
18. Cabbage, onion, carrot miso soup 1b. Pressure-cooked brown rice 49. Rice cream 216. Zucchini, onion nitsuke 137. Cabbage, celery nuka pickles	**Sunday, September 9**	1b. Pressure-cooked brown rice 60. Vegetable oden 260. French-fried potatoes 261. Goma tofu 137. Cucumber nuka pickles
18. Turnip, beet, onion miso soup 1b. Pressure-cooked brown rice 32. Kidney beans with miso 227a. String bean, onion, celery nitsuke 137. Cucumber, cabbage nuka pickles	**Monday, September 10**	1b. Pressure-cooked brown rice 253,38. Togan with kuzu sauce *and* Kasha croquettes (leftover) 148. Hijiki nori nitsuke 137. Celery, cabbage nuka pickles
18. Wakame, onion, cabbage, carrot miso soup 1b. Pressure-cooked brown rice 49. Rice cream 34. Butternut squash, onion nitsuke 137. Daikon, celery nuka pickles	**Tuesday, September 11**	1b. Pressure-cooked brown rice 24,25. Kasha *with* Sesame sauce 251. Pan-fried eggplant with miso 137. Daikon, cucumber nuka pickles

Breakfast		*Dinner*
28. Wakame, onion, cabbage, carrot miso soup 1b. Pressure-cooked brown rice 49. Rice cream 19. Bok choy, onion, carrot nitsuke 64. Home-made age 23. Grated daikon 137. Cabbage, celery nuka pickles	**Wednesday, September 12**	*Dinner for Non-Macrobiotic Parents* 1b. Pressure-cooked brown rice 262,187. Fried quail *with* Curry sauce (similar) 114. Saifun salad 148. Hijiki nori nitsuke 263a. Parsley miso pickles 132. Amasake cake with yannoh frosting
18. Cabbage, onion, carrot miso soup 1b. Pressure-cooked brown rice 136. Oatmeal 140. Dried daikon nitsuke 13. Natto with pickled daikon leaves 137. Cabbage, celery nuka pickles	**Thursday, September 13**	1b. Pressure-cooked brown rice 50. Millet with chick pea sauce 257. Green pepper with sauteed miso 189. Corn bread 137. Cabbage, celery nuka pickles
18. Cabbage, onion, carrot miso soup 1a. Azuki bean rice 208. Corn meal 227a,64. String bean, Chinese cabbage nitsuke (similar) *with* Home-made age 137. Daikon, cabbage nuka pickles	**Friday, September 14**	1b. Pressure-cooked brown rice 47. Cauliflower, string bean, onion, carrot with kuzu sauce (similar) 30. Nori nitsuke 137. Cabbage, celery nuka pickles
18. Daikon, burdock, onion, carrot miso soup 1b. Pressure-cooked brown rice 49. Rice cream 216. Zucchini, onion nitsuke 137. Chinese cabbage, daikon nuka pickles	**Saturday, September 15**	1b. Pressure-cooked brown rice 264,187. Kasha - potato croquettes *with* Curry sauce (similar) 114. Saifun salad (leftover) 241a. Corn on the cob 137. Celery nuka pickles
18. Daikon, burdock, onion, carrot miso soup 1b. Pressure-cooked brown rice 241a. Corn on the cob 137. Daikon nuka pickles	**Sunday, September 16**	1b. Pressure-cooked brown rice 187,50. Curry sauce (leftover) *with* Millet 123. Cabbage roll with bonita flakes

Breakfast		*Dinner*
Wedding Menu – see also dinner column 1a. Azuki bean rice 265. Matsuba kombu 123. Chinese cabbage spiral roll 114. Saifun salad 7. Yam - chestnut kinton 266. Amasake wedding cake 90. Oatmeal cookies 267. Musubi kombu 268. Shad with tomato sauce	**Sunday, September 16** *(continued)* Wedding Menu Served early afternoon	*Wedding Menu continued* 269. Bamboo roll 270. Fuku musubi 146. Norimake sushi 249. Peach kanten (similar) 271. Apple juice with bancha tea Corn chips Rice cakes Watermelon Champagne
18. Chinese cabbage, onion, carrot miso soup 1b. Pressure-cooked brown rice 49. Rice cream 55. Cabbage nitsuke 137. Cucumber nuka pickles	**Monday, September 17**	1b. Pressure-cooked brown rice 264,25. Kasha croquettes (leftover) *with* Sesame onion sauce 66. Spinach ohitashi with bonita flakes 137. Cucumber, celery nuka pickles
18. Chinese cabbage, onion, carrot miso soup 1b. Pressure-cooked brown rice 13. Natto with pickled daikon leaves 49. Rice cream 186. Hijiki nitsuke 137. Cucumber, celery nuka pickles	**Tuesday, September 18**	*Cooking Class* 41. Baked rice 272. Azuki bean stew with bread 30. Nori nitsuke 273. Onion soup 231. Cabbage pressed salad
18. Bok choy, onion, carrot miso soup 1b. Pressure-cooked brown rice 49. Rice cream 55. Cabbage, onion, carrot nitsuke (similar) 137. Chinese cabbage nuka pickles	**Wednesday, September 19**	1b. Pressure-cooked brown rice 29. Pan-fried whole wheat spaghetti 47. Vegetables with kuzu sauce (similar) 137. Cucumber, cabbage nuka pickles
18. Cabbage, onion, carrot miso soup 1b. Pressure-cooked brown rice 55. Cabbage nitsuke (leftover) 13. Natto with pickled daikon leaves 15. Chinese cabbage nuka pickles	**Thursday, September 20**	274. Shingiku miso soup 149. Ohagi with green pea, chestnut, sesame seeds, baked nori toppings 36. Vegetable gratin 137. Daikon, cucumber nuka pickles

Breakfast		*Dinner*
274. Shingiku and dried fu miso soup 1b. Pressure-cooked brown rice 208. Corn meal 54. Broccoli nitsuke 137. Daikon, celery nuka pickles	**Friday, September 21**	1b. Pressure-cooked brown rice 151. Stuffed cabbage with white sauce 257. Green pepper with sauteed miso 21a,143. Tossed salad *with* Umeboshi dressing 249. Fruit kanten
18. Cabbage, onion, carrot miso soup 1b. Pressure-cooked brown rice 49. Rice cream 216. Crookneck squash, zucchini nitsuke 15. Chinese cabbage nuka pickles	**Saturday, September 22**	119. Fried rice 29. Fried spaghetti (leftover) 75. Northern white beans with white miso 21a. Watermelon salad (similar)
18. Cabbage, onion, carrot miso soup 1b. Pressure-cooked brown rice 49. Rice cream 19. Collard green, onion, carrot nitsuke 137. Watermelon rind, cabbage nuka pickles	**Sunday, September 23**	1b. Pressure-cooked brown rice 22a. Vegetable tempura 122. Tempura sauce with ginger 26. Boiled beets 31. Apple pie
28. Wakame, onion, cabbage, carrot miso soup 1b. Pressure-cooked brown rice 136. Oatmeal 216. Squash nitsuke with shingiku 137. Watermelon rind, cabbage nuka pickles	**Monday, September 24**	1b. Pressure-cooked brown rice 222,191a. Somen with tomato sauce 275. Baked stuffed zucchini 276. Kombu - egg nitsuke 15. Chinese cabbage nuka pickles
18. Turnip, onion, string bean, carrot miso soup 1b. Pressure-cooked brown rice 136. Green vegetable nitsuke 141. Condiment pickles	**Tuesday, September 25**	*Cooking Class* 1b. Pressure-cooked brown rice 277. Garlic fried rice 186. Hijiki nitsuke 278. Carrot nitsuke 197. Onion cream miso soup
18. Turnip, onion, string bean, leek miso soup 1b. Pressure-cooked brown rice 49. Rice cream 34. Butternut squash, onion nitsuke 137. Celery, cabbage nuka pickles	**Wednesday, September 26**	1b. Pressure-cooked brown rice 24,25. Kasha *with* Sesame sauce 26. Boiled beets 137. Cucumber, celery nuka pickles

Breakfast		Dinner
18,75. Miso soup (leftover) *mixed with* Northern white beans with miso (leftover) 1b. Pressure-cooked brown rice 13. Natto with pickled daikon leaves 137. Cabbage, celery nuka pickles	**Thursday, September 27**	*Herman's Birthday Dinner* 134. Gomoku rice 138. Vegetable kebabs with lemon miso sauce 279. Buckwheat potage with croutons 132. Amasake cake
18,279. Scallion miso soup *mixed with* Buckwheat potage (leftover) 1b. Pressure-cooked brown rice 49. Rice cream 227a. String bean nitsuke 14,15. Daikon, cabbage nuka pickles	**Friday, September 28**	222,191a. Somen *with* Tomato sauce 66. Swiss chard ohitashi with bonita flakes 14,15. Daikon, cabbage nuka pickles
18. Cabbage, onion, carrot miso soup 1b. Pressure-cooked brown rice 32. Kidney beans with miso 15. Chinese cabbage nuka pickles	**Saturday, September 29**	1b. Pressure-cooked brown rice 280. Fried chicken wings 91. Saifun nitsuke 21a. Tossed salad
18. Swiss chard, onion, carrot miso soup 1b. Pressure-cooked brown rice 216. Zucchini nitsuke 13. Natto with pickled daikon leaves 49. Rice cream 15. Chinese cabbage nuka pickles	**Sunday, September 30**	1b. Pressure-cooked brown rice 253. Togan and onion with kuzu sauce 148. Hijiki nori nitsuke 241a. Corn on the cob 14,15. Daikon, cabbage nuka pickles

October

Breakfast		Dinner
1a. Azuki bean rice 18. Swiss chard, onion, carrot miso soup 35. Onion miso 14,15. Daikon, cabbage nuka pickles	**Monday, October 1**	1b. Pressure-cooked brown rice 281. Fresh corn with onion cream sauce 282. Konnyaku nitsuke 15. Chinese cabbage nuka pickles
32,18. Kidney beans with vegetable miso soup 1b. Pressure-cooked brown rice 216. Zucchini nitsuke 141. Condiment pickles	**Tuesday, October 2**	*Cooking Class* 62. Sakura rice 127. Squash potage with croutons 154. Vegetable macaroni stew 283. Puri 21a. Tossed salad
28. Wakame, onion, cabbage, carrot miso soup 1b. Pressure-cooked brown rice 49. Rice cream 70. Sauteed cabbage and bean sprouts 137. Daikon nuka pickles	**Wednesday, October 3**	24,25. Kasha *with* Sesame sauce 91. Saifun nitsuke 15. Chinese cabbage nuka pickles
28. Wakame, onion, cabbage, carrot miso soup 1b. Pressure-cooked brown rice 155. Burdock, onion, carrot fritters 136. Oatmeal 137. Cabbage, celery nuka pickles	**Thursday, October 4**	1b. Pressure-cooked brown rice 50. Millet with chick pea sauce 284. Shingiku goma ai 170,152. Rice bread *with* Apple butter 15. Chinese cabbage nuka pickles
18. Cabbage, onion, carrot miso soup 1b. Pressure-cooked brown rice 49. Rice cream 154. Vegetable macaroni stew (leftover) 14. Chinese cabbage nuka pickles	**Friday, October 5**	1b. Pressure-cooked brown rice 74. Uosuki 214. Rice salad 15. Chinese cabbage nuka pickles

Breakfast		Dinner
18. Chinese cabbage, onion, carrot miso soup 1b. Pressure-cooked brown rice 136. Oatmeal 17. Chick pea sauce 15. Chinese cabbage nuka pickles	**Saturday, October 6**	1b. Pressure-cooked brown rice 38,37. Kasha croquettes *with* Onion bechamel sauce 66. Shingiku ohitashi 15. Chinese cabbage nuka pickles
18. Chinese cabbage, onion, carrot miso soup 1b. Pressure-cooked brown rice 91. Saifun nitsuke 15. Chinese cabbage nuka pickles	**Sunday, October 7**	1b. Pressure-cooked brown rice 191. Sesame spaghetti with tomato sauce 148. Hijiki nori nitsuke 15. Chinese cabbage nuka pickles
18. Daikon, scallion, carrot miso soup 1b. Pressure-cooked brown rice 136. Oatmeal 13. Natto with pickled daikon leaves 137. Cabbage, celery nuka pickles	**Monday, October 8**	1b. Pressure-cooked brown rice 138. Boiled cabbage, cauliflower 120. Wild pigeon shish-kebab 15. Chinese cabbage nuka pickles
18. Daikon, scallion, carrot miso soup 1b. Pressure-cooked brown rice 49. Rice cream 54. Broccoli nitsuke 15. Chinese cabbage nuka pickles	**Tuesday, October 9**	*Cooking Class* 1b. Pressure-cooked brown rice 80a,87b. Clear soup *with* Dried fu 285. Udon with mock meat sauce 140. Dried daikon nitsuke 190. Apple - chestnut ring
18. Daikon, scallion, carrot miso soup 1b. Pressure-cooked brown rice 19. Takana, onion nitsuke (similar) 136. Oatmeal 15. Chinese cabbage nuka pickles	**Wednesday, October 10**	1b. Pressure-cooked brown rice 110. Vegetable stew 71. Azuki winter squash nitsuke 72. Kombu nori nitsuke 14. Daikon nuka pickles
18. Leek, turnip, carrot miso soup 1b. Pressure-cooked brown rice 136. Oatmeal 36. Vegetable nitsuke (leftover) casserole 15. Chinese cabbage nuka pickles	**Thursday, October 11**	1b. Pressure-cooked brown rice 176. Lentil soup 65,37. Millet burgers *with* Bechamel sauce 286. Shingiku, endive norimake 15. Chinese cabbage nuka pickles

Breakfast		*Dinner*
18. Leek, turnip, carrot miso soup 1b. Pressure-cooked brown rice 140,22c. Dried daikon nitsuke *with* Tempura crumbs 13. Natto with pickled daikon leaves	**Friday, October 12**	1b. Pressure-cooked brown rice 29. Pan-fried whole wheat spaghetti 30. Nori nitsuke 286. Shingiku, endive norimake 15. Chinese cabbage nuka pickles
Mirimichi Camp begins 287. Pan-fried mochi with nori 125,126. Rice balls *with* Shio kombu 176. Lentil soup with miso 65. Millet burgers 15. Chinese cabbage nuka pickles	**Saturday, October 13**	1b. Pressure-cooked brown rice 24,25. Kasha *with* Sesame sauce 125. Rice balls 175. Daikon top and broccoli nitsuke 14. Daikon nuka pickles
1a. Azuki bean rice 28. Wakame, onion, cabbage, carrot miso soup 55. Cabbage nitsuke 14. Daikon nuka pickles	**Sunday, October 14**	1b. Pressure-cooked brown rice 110. Vegetable stew 97. Scallion miso 21a. Tossed green salad
52. Vegetable ojiya 155. Burdock, onion, carrot fritters 14. Daikon nuka pickles	**Monday, October 15**	1b. Pressure-cooked brown rice 288. Buckwheat macaroni soup 275. Stuffed zucchini squash 15. Chinese cabbage nuka pickles 31. Apple pie
52. Butternut squash, onion ojiya 289. Burdock, carrot, fresh mushroom nitsuke 137. Daikon top, cabbage, cucumber nuka pickles	**Tuesday, October 16**	1b. Pressure-cooked brown rice 50. Millet with chick pea sauce 30. Nori nitsuke 15. Chinese cabbage nuka pickles
18. Turnip, onion, carrot miso soup 1b. Pressure-cooked brown rice 216. Zucchini nitsuke 15. Chinese cabbage nuka pickles	**Wednesday, October 17**	*George Ohsawa's Birthday Dinner* 1b. Pressure-cooked brown rice 2B. Steamed mochi 2a. Mochi soup 2b. Azuki squash mochi 2c. Walnut mochi 66. Ohitashi

Breakfast		*Dinner*
18. Onion, zucchini, carrot miso soup 1b. Pressure-cooked brown rice 221. Hijiki, carrot, carrot top nitsuke 15. Chinese cabbage nuka pickles	**Thursday, October 18**	1b. Pressure-cooked brown rice 288. Buckwheat macaroni soup 257. Green pepper with oily miso 14. Daikon nuka pickles
18. Beet, onion, carrot miso soup 1b. Pressure-cooked brown rice 34. Squash and onion nitsuke 14. Daikon nuka pickles	**Friday, October 19**	1b. Pressure-cooked brown rice 290. Tofu with kuzu sauce 150. Sweet potato, parsnip nitsuke 14. Daikon nuka pickles 31. Apple pie
18. Wakame, onion, carrot miso soup 1b. Pressure-cooked brown rice 100. Okara nitsuke 14. Daikon nuka pickles	**Saturday, October 20**	1b. Pressure-cooked brown rice 127. Pumpkin potage with croutons 91. Saifun nitsuke 15. Chinese cabbage nuka pickles
1b. Pressure-cooked brown rice 125. Rice balls 100. Okara nitsuke (leftover) 14. Daikon nuka pickles *Mirimichi Camp ends*	**Sunday, October 21**	1b. Pressure-cooked brown rice 53. Clear soup with noodles 14,15. Daikon, cabbage nuka pickles
18. Squash, onion, bok choy miso soup 1b. Pressure-cooked brown rice 75. Northern white beans with miso 13. Natto with pickled daikon leaves 15. Chinese cabbage nuka pickles	**Monday, October 22**	1b. Pressure-cooked brown rice 291. Noodle sukiyaki 221. Hijiki carrot nitsuke 14,15. Daikon, cabbage nuka pickles
28. Wakame, onion, cabbage, carrot miso soup 1b. Pressure-cooked brown rice 34. Squash and onion nitsuke 14,15. Daikon, cabbage nuka pickles 31. Apple pie	**Tuesday, October 23**	*Cooking Class* 1b. Pressure-cooked brown rice 292. Whole wheat bread 80b. Tofu, watercress white miso soup 91. Saifun nitsuke 14. Daikon nuka pickles 293. Apricot kanten

Breakfast		*Dinner*
28. Wakame, onion, cabbage, carrot miso soup 1b. Pressure-cooked brown rice 331. Toasted nori 86. Fresh daikon nitsuke 15. Chinese cabbage nuka pickles	**Wednesday, October 24**	1b. Pressure-cooked brown rice 47. Cauliflower with kuzu sauce 221. Hijiki carrot nitsuke (leftover) 14,15. Daikon, cabbage nuka pickles
18. Turnip, onion, carrot miso soup 1b. Pressure-cooked brown rice 13. Natto with pickled daikon leaves 75,34. White beans *mixed with* Squash and onion nitsuke (leftover) 15. Chinese cabbage nuka pickles	**Thursday, October 25**	1b. Pressure-cooked brown rice 110. Vegetable stew 294. Soybean nitsuke 15. Chinese cabbage nuka pickles
18. Turnip, onion, carrot miso soup 1b. Pressure-cooked brown rice 85. Chinese cabbage, onion, carrot nitsuke 14. Daikon nuka pickles	**Friday, October 26**	1b. Pressure-cooked brown rice 295. Baked fresh tuna 91. Saifun nitsuke 15. Chinese cabbage nuka pickles
18. Turnip, onion, carrot miso soup 1b. Pressure-cooked brown rice 54. Broccoli nitsuke 15. Chinese cabbage nuka pickles	**Saturday, October 27**	62. Sakura rice 60. Vegetable oden 61. Green pea nitsuke 15. Chinese cabbage nuka pickles 296. Apple butter kanten
18. Turnip, onion, carrot miso soup 1b. Pressure-cooked brown rice 83,152. Waffles with maple syrup, butter *and* Home-made apple butter 100. Okara nitsuke 15. Chinese cabbage nuka pickles	**Sunday, October 28**	1b. Pressure-cooked brown rice 110. Vegetable stew (leftover) 21a. Tossed salad 141. Condiment pickles
18. Cabbage, onion, carrot miso soup 1b. Pressure-cooked brown rice 49. Rice cream 63. Collard green, onion, cabbage, age nitsuke 15. Chinese cabbage nuka pickles	**Monday, October 29**	1b. Pressure-cooked brown rice 29,37. Fried buckwheat noodles *with* Bechamel sauce 66. Shingiku, mustard green ohitashi with kirigoma 15. Chinese cabbage nuka pickles

Breakfast		Dinner
18. Cabbage, onion, carrot miso soup 1b. Pressure-cooked brown rice 71. Azuki squash nitsuke 91. Saifun nitsuke (leftover) 15. Chinese cabbage nuka pickles	**Tuesday, October 30**	*Cooking Class* 1b. Pressure-cooked brown rice 297. Chick pea with sweet brown rice 115. Egg drop soup 103. Vegetables with tahini sauce 132. Amasake cake with yannoh frosting 14. Daikon nuka pickles
18. Bok choy, onion, butternut squash miso soup 1b. Pressure-cooked brown rice 60. Oden (leftover) 14,15. Daikon, cabbage nuka pickles	**Wednesday, October 31**	119,37. Fried rice *with* Bechamel sauce 102. Buckwheat noodle casserole 21a. Tossed salad 143. Umeboshi, onion, orange rind dressing

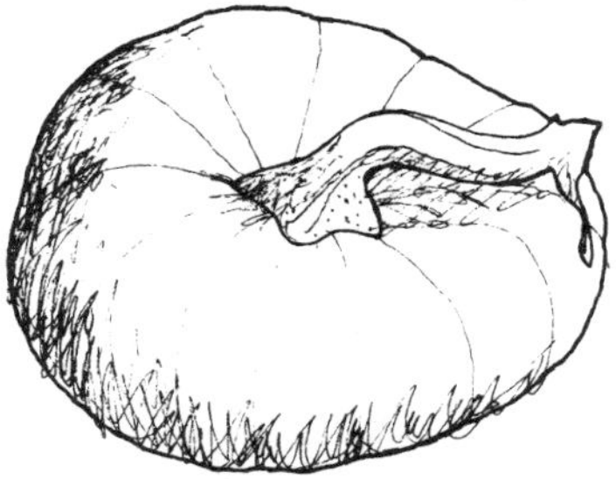

November

Breakfast		Dinner
18. Bok choy, onion, butternut squash miso soup 1a. Azuki bean rice 298. Dandelion root, burdock nitsuke 15. Chinese cabbage nuka pickles	**Thursday, November 1**	1b. Pressure-cooked brown rice 288. Buckwheat macaroni soup 34. Winter squash, onion nitsuke 72. Nori kombu nitsuke 15. Chinese cabbage nuka pickles
18,288. Miso soup *mixed with* Macaroni soup 1b. Pressure-cooked brown rice 49. Rice cream 35. Onion miso 15. Takana, Chinese cabbage nuka pickles	**Friday, November 2**	1b. Pressure-cooked brown rice 84,37. Rice and noodle burger *with* Bechamel sauce 15. Chinese cabbage nuka pickles
18. Daikon, onion, carrot miso soup 1b. Pressure-cooked brown rice 91. Saifun nitsuke 299. Scallion condiment	**Saturday, November 3**	1b. Pressure-cooked brown rice 50. Millet with chick pea sauce 103. Lettuce with tahini sauce 15. Chinese cabbage nuka pickles 31. Apple pie
18. Daikon, onion, carrot miso soup 1b. Pressure-cooked brown rice 54. Broccoli nitsuke 14,15. Daikon, cabbage nuka pickles	**Sunday, November 4**	*Invited Out.*
18. Swiss chard, onion, carrot miso soup 1b. Pressure-cooked brown rice 50,91,54. Nitsuke made from leftovers 13. Natto with pickled daikon leaves 15. Chinese cabbage nuka pickles	**Monday, November 5**	1b. Pressure-cooked brown rice 110. Vegetable stew 72. Nori kombu nitsuke 15. Chinese cabbage nuka pickles
18. Swiss chard, onion, carrot miso soup 1b. Pressure-cooked brown rice 34. Winter squash, onion nitsuke 14,15. Daikon, cabbage nuka pickles	**Tuesday, November 6**	*Cooking Class* 18. Daikon, onion, carrot miso soup 1b. Pressure-cooked brown rice 22a,122. Vegetable tempura *with* Tempura sauce 108. Squash bread 15. Chinese cabbage nuka pickles 301. Sauteed apples and pumpkin

Breakfast			Dinner	
18.	Daikon, onion, carrot miso soup	**Wednesday, November 7**	1b.	Pressure-cooked brown rice
1b.	Pressure-cooked brown rice		32.	Pinto beans with miso (similar)
294.	Soybean nitsuke		302.	Parsnip, beet nitsuke
14,15.	Daikon, cabbage nuka pickles		15.	Chinese cabbage nuka pickles
18.	Cabbage, onion, carrot miso soup	**Thursday, November 8**	1b.	Pressure-cooked brown rice
1b.	Pressure-cooked brown rice		303.	Stuffed acorn squash
34.	Winter squash, onion nitsuke		304.	Kombu, dried tofu, age nitsuke
14,15.	Daikon, cabbage nuka pickles		305b.	Millet soup
			15.	Chinese cabbage nuka pickles
18,305a.	Miso soup *and* Millet soup	**Friday, November 9**	1b.	Pressure-cooked brown rice
1b.	Pressure-cooked brown rice		29.	Pan-fried whole wheat spaghetti
36.	Casserole made from leftover nitsuke		26.	Boiled beets
15.	Chinese cabbage nuka pickles		15.	Chinese cabbage nuka pickles
			306.	Vegetable raisin pie
18.	Chinese cabbage, onion, carrot miso soup	**Saturday, November 10**	1b.	Pressure-cooked brown rice
1b.	Pressure-cooked brown rice		130.	Rice pie
71.	Azuki squash nitsuke		21a.	Tossed salad
276.	Kombu nitsuke (similar)		71.	Azuki squash nitsuke (leftover)
15.	Chinese cabbage nuka pickles			
18.	Daikon, onion, tofu miso soup	**Sunday, November 11**	1b.	Pressure-cooked brown rice
1b.	Pressure-cooked brown rice		53.	Whole wheat noodles with broth
307.	Wild scallion nitsuke		130.	Rice pie
15.	Chinese cabbage nuka pickles		58.	French bread
			15.	Chinese cabbage nuka pickles
18.	Winter squash, onion miso soup	**Monday, November 12**	1b.	Pressure-cooked brown rice
1b.	Pressure-cooked brown rice		24,25.	Kasha *with* Sesame sauce
13.	Natto with pickled daikon leaves		72.	Nori kombu nitsuke
71.	Azuki squash nitsuke (leftover)		303.	Stuffed acorn squash (leftover)
141.	Condiment pickles		15.	Chinese cabbage nuka pickles

Breakfast		Dinner
18. Winter squash, onion miso soup 1b. Pressure-cooked brown rice 57. Carrot, carrot-top with sesame seed nitsuke 263b. Shiso seed miso pickles	**Tuesday, November 13**	*Cooking Class* 1b. Pressure-cooked brown rice 305b. Millet soup 308. Vegetable pie 30. Nori nitsuke 14. Daikon nuka pickles 193. Tahini custard
305b. Millet soup with miso 1b. Pressure-cooked brown rice 307. Wild scallion and seitan nitsuke 276. Kombu nitsuke with sesame seeds 15. Chinese cabbage nuka pickles	**Wednesday, November 14**	1b. Pressure-cooked brown rice 2C. Mugwort mochi 2a. Mochi soup 2b. Azuki - squash mochi 2c. Walnut mochi 294. Soybean nitsuke 66. Swiss chard ohitashi with roasted white sesame seeds 90. Daikon pressed salad
18. Collard green, onion, carrot miso soup 1b. Pressure-cooked brown rice 86. Fresh daikon nitsuke 2b. Azuki - squash mochi (leftover) 15. Chinese cabbage nuka pickles	**Thursday, November 15**	1b. Pressure-cooked brown rice 47. Cauliflower with kuzu sauce 257. Green pepper with sauteed miso 14. Daikon top nuka pickles
18. Collard green, onion, carrot miso soup 1b. Pressure-cooked brown rice 34. Squash, onion, bok choy nitsuke 15. Chinese cabbage nuka pickles	**Friday, November 16**	1b. Pressure-cooked brown rice 38,37. Kasha croquettes *with* Bechamel sauce 309. Steamed cabbage 14. Daikon nuka pickles
18. Squash, onion, bok choy miso soup 1b. Pressure-cooked brown rice 54. Broccoli nitsuke 14. Daikon nuka pickles	**Saturday, November 17**	1b. Pressure-cooked brown rice 2a. Mochi soup with scallion and watercress 308. Vegetable pie 276. Kombu nitsuke 14. Daikon nuka pickles
Gone for entire day.	**Sunday, November 18**	*Gone for entire day.*

Breakfast		Dinner
18. Cabbage, onion, carrot miso soup 1b. Pressure-cooked brown rice 278. Carrot nitsuke 13. Natto with pickled daikon leaves 14,15. Daikon, cabbage nuka pickles	**Monday, November 19**	1b. Pressure-cooked brown rice 53. Udon with tempura 22a. Tempura 14,15. Daikon, cabbage nuka pickles
18,29. Miso soup (leftover) *mixed with* Fried noodles (leftover) 1b. Pressure-cooked brown rice 307. Scallion, celery nitsuke (similar) 14,15. Daikon, cabbage nuka pickles	**Tuesday, November 20**	*Cooking Class* 1b. Pressure-cooked brown rice 129. Clear party soup with vegetables 24,25. Kasha *with* Sesame sauce 133. Sweet potato, carrot nitsuke 292. Whole wheat bread 310a,b,c. Cranberry sauce
18. Turnip, onion, carrot miso soup 1b. Pressure-cooked brown rice 311. Lotus root nitsuke 137. Chinese cabbage, celery nuka pickles	**Wednesday, November 21**	1b. Pressure-cooked brown rice 29,37. Pan-fried noodles and parsley *with* Bechamel sauce 300. Turnip, turnip top nitsuke (similar) 312,310a. Whole wheat buns *with* Cranberry sauce
Special Day – one meal only.	**Thursday, November 22**	*Thanksgiving Dinner* 41. Baked rice 166. Roast turkey with stuffing 80a. Clear soup with tofu and shingiku 313. Brussels sprouts - beet salad with mayonnaise dressing 77,166a. Mashed potatoes *with* Gravy 76. Macaroni salad 81,310a. White buns *with* Cranberry sauce 314. Pumpkin pie 315. Tangerine kanten
18. Daikon, onion, Brussels sprouts leaves miso soup 1b. Pressure-cooked brown rice 300. Mustard green and onion nitsuke 15. Chinese cabbage nuka pickles	**Friday, November 23**	1b. Pressure-cooked brown rice 53. Udon with clear broth 313. Cooked salad (leftover) 276. Kombu nitsuke (leftover) 14. Daikon nuka pickles

Breakfast		*Dinner*
18. Miso soup with watercress (leftover) 1b. Pressure-cooked brown rice 32. Pinto beans with miso 15. Chinese cabbage nuka pickles	**Saturday, November 24**	1b. Pressure-cooked brown rice 60. Vegetable oden 15. Chinese cabbage nuka pickles
18. Turnip, turnip top, leek, carrot miso soup 1b. Pressure-cooked brown rice 83,152, 310a. Waffles *with* Apple butter *and* Cranberry sauce 14. Daikon nuka pickles	**Sunday, November 25**	*Dinner Out.*
18. Turnip, onion, turnip top, carrot miso soup 1b. Pressure-cooked brown rice 34. Winter squash and onion nitsuke 141. Condiment pickles	**Monday, November 26**	1b. Pressure-cooked brown rice 60. Oden (leftover) 66. Swiss chard ohitashi 132. Amasake cake
18. Turnip, turnip top, leek, carrot miso soup 1b. Pressure-cooked brown rice 300. New Zealand spinach and Swiss chard nitsuke (similar) 14. Daikon, daikon top nuka pickles	**Tuesday, November 27**	*Cooking Class* 1b. Pressure-cooked brown rice 118. Baked squash with sesame sauce 316. Country potage 317. Watercress nitsuke 15. Chinese cabbage nuka pickles 124. Apple crisp
80b. Tofu - watercress miso soup (similar) 1b. Pressure-cooked brown rice 72. Nori nitsuke with leftover kombu 32. Pinto beans with miso (leftover) 14. Daikon nuka pickles	**Wednesday, November 28**	1b. Pressure-cooked brown rice 38,37. Kasha croquettes *with* Bechamel sauce 66. New Zealand spinach and shingiku ohitashi with bonita flakes, kirigoma 15. Chinese cabbage nuka pickles
18. Wakame, onion, cabbage, carrot miso soup 1b. Pressure-cooked brown rice 66. Ohitashi (leftover) made into nitsuke 14. Daikon nuka pickles	**Thursday, November 29**	1b. Pressure-cooked brown rice 318. Stuffed green peppers (made with leftover turkey stuffing) 30. Nori nitsuke 14. Daikon nuka pickles

Breakfast		*Dinner*
28. Wakame, onion, carrot, cabbage miso soup 1a. Azuki bean rice 43. Burdock, carrot kinpira 14. Daikon nuka pickles	**Friday, November 30**	1b. Pressure-cooked brown rice 71. Pinto beans with yam nitsuke (similar) 54. Broccoli nitsuke 14. Daikon nuka pickles

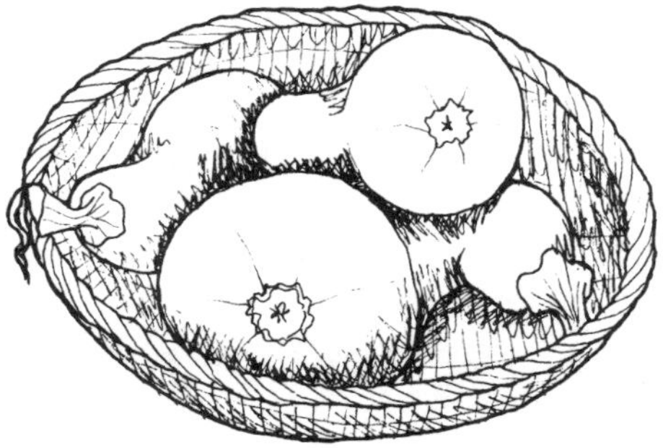

December

Breakfast / *Dinner*

Saturday, December 1

Breakfast

18. Burdock, daikon, carrot miso soup
1b. Pressure-cooked brown rice
55. Cabbage nitsuke
14. Daikon nuka pickles

Dinner

1b. Pressure-cooked brown rice
29. Pan-fried whole wheat spaghetti
26. Boiled beets
15. Chinese cabbage nuka pickles

Sunday, December 2

Breakfast

18. Burdock, daikon, carrot miso soup
1b. Pressure-cooked brown rice
64. Fried tofu
23. Grated daikon, carrot
14. Daikon nuka pickles

Dinner

1b. Pressure-cooked brown rice
36,166,77. Gratin *made from* Turkey stuffing (leftover) *and* Mashed potato (leftover)
72. Nori kombu nitsuke
15. Chinese cabbage nuka pickles
319. Currant kanten

Monday, December 3

Breakfast

18,28. Squash, onion miso soup *with* Steamed mochi
1b. Pressure-cooked brown rice
85. Chinese cabbage, onion, carrot nitsuke
97. Scallion miso
137. Jerusalem artichoke, Chinese cabbage nuka pickles

Dinner

1b. Pressure-cooked brown rice
24,25. Kasha *with* Sesame sauce
61. Green pea nitsuke
319. Kanten (leftover)
15. Chinese cabbage nuka pickles

Tuesday, December 4

Breakfast

18,29. Squash, onion miso soup *with* Fried spaghetti (leftover)
1b. Pressure-cooked brown rice
55. Cabbage nitsuke
14. Daikon, daikon top nuka pickles

Dinner

Cooking Class

134. Gomoku rice
80a. Clear soup with dried fu
123. Chinese cabbage roll
320. Cucumber mustard pickles with amasake
7. Yam - chestnut kinton

Wednesday, December 5

Breakfast

18,2C. Squash, onion miso soup *with* Mugwort mochi
1b. Pressure-cooked brown rice
321. Cracked wheat with onions
54. Burdock, carrot kinpira
14. Daikon nuka pickles

Dinner

1b. Pressure-cooked brown rice
36,61, 24,37. Casserole *made from* Green pea nitsuke *and* Kasha *with* Bechamel sauce
51. Hijiki, lotus root nitsuke
56. Garlic French bread
15. Chinese cabbage nuka pickles

Breakfast		Dinner
18. Daikon, onion, carrot miso soup 1b. Pressure-cooked brown rice 54. Broccoli nitsuke 97. Scallion miso 14,15. Daikon, cabbage nuka pickles	**Thursday, December 6**	322. Baked rice with seitan and walnuts 91. Saifun nitsuke 127. Pumpkin potage with croutons 15. Chinese cabbage nuka pickles
18,2C. Daikon, onion, carrot miso soup *with* Mugwort mochi 1b. Pressure-cooked brown rice 140. Dried daikon nitsuke 15. Chinese cabbage nuka pickles	**Friday, December 7**	1b. Pressure-cooked brown rice 47. Cauliflower with kuzu sauce 51. Hijiki, lotus root nitsuke 15. Chinese cabbage nuka pickles
18. Cauliflower leaves, onion, carrot miso soup 1b. Pressure-cooked brown rice 32. Kidney beans with miso 15. Chinese cabbage nuka pickles	**Saturday, December 8**	1b. Pressure-cooked brown rice 323,37. Rice patties *with* Bechamel sauce 66. Swiss chard ohitashi 15. Chinese cabbage nuka pickles
18. Cauliflower leaves, onion, carrot miso soup 1b. Pressure-cooked brown rice 324. Turnip, turnip top and sake-kasu nitsuke with chirimen iriko 15. Chinese cabbage nuka pickles	**Sunday, December 9**	80b. Tofu - scallion miso soup 1b. Pressure-cooked brown rice 325. Fried oysters with fried saifun 15. Chinese cabbage nuka pickles 319. Dried fruits kanten (similar)
80b. Tofu - scallion miso soup 1b. Pressure-cooked brown rice 91. Saifun nitsuke (leftover) 141,16a. Condiment pickles *with* Roasted nori	**Monday, December 10**	1b. Pressure-cooked brown rice 50. Millet with chick pea sauce 148. Hijiki nori nitsuke 15. Chinese cabbage nuka pickles
18. Cabbage, onion, carrot miso soup 1b. Pressure-cooked brown rice 300. Mustard green and onion nitsuke 15. Chinese cabbage nuka pickles	**Tuesday, December 11**	*Cooking Class* 2a. Mochi soup 2C. Mugwort mochi 2b. Azuki squash mochi 2c. Walnut mochi 327. Kombu roll 14. Daikon nuka pickles

Breakfast		Dinner
18. Cabbage, onion, carrot miso soup 1b. Pressure-cooked brown rice 324,140, 36,37. Turnip, dried daikon nitsuke (leftover) gratin *with* Bechamel sauce and bread crumbs 137. Mustard green nuka pickles	**Wednesday, December 12**	*Dinner Out.*
18,2b,c. Cabbage, onion, carrot miso soup *with* Azuki squash *and* Walnut mochi 1b. Pressure-cooked brown rice 17. Chick pea sauce (leftover) 14. Daikon nuka pickles	**Thursday, December 13**	1b. Pressure-cooked brown rice 40. Russian soup 140. Dried daikon nitsuke 15. Chinese cabbage nuka pickles 135. Amasake doughnuts
1a. Azuki bean rice 2a,40. Mochi soup *mixed with* Russian soup 327. Kombu roll (leftover) 14. Daikon nuka pickles	**Friday, December 14**	1b. Pressure-cooked brown rice 47. Cauliflower with kuzu sauce 30. Nori nitsuke 141. Condiment pickles
18. Bok choy, onion, carrot miso soup 1b. Pressure-cooked brown rice 2b. Azuki mochi (leftover) 91. Saifun nitsuke 14. Daikon nuka pickles	**Saturday, December 15**	1b. Pressure-cooked brown rice 24,25. Kasha *with* Sesame sauce 328. Parsnip, watercress nitsuke 14,15. Daikon, cabbage nuka pickles
18. Bok choy, onion, carrot miso soup 1b. Pressure-cooked brown rice 32. Kidney beans with miso 15. Chinese cabbage nuka pickles	**Sunday, December 16**	1b. Pressure-cooked brown rice 47. Cauliflower with kuzu sauce (leftover) 30. Nori nitsuke (leftover) 14. Daikon nuka pickles 329. Amasake crescent cookies
18. Squash, onion miso soup 1b. Pressure-cooked brown rice 140. Dried daikon nitsuke 14. Daikon nuka pickles	**Monday, December 17**	1b. Pressure-cooked brown rice 40. Russian soup (leftover) with watercress 32. Kidney beans with miso 56. Garlic bread 15. Chinese cabbage nuka pickles

Breakfast		Dinner
18. Squash, onion miso soup 1b. Pressure-cooked brown rice 155. Burdock, onion, carrot fritters 15. Chinese cabbage nuka pickles	**Tuesday, December 18**	1b. Pressure-cooked brown rice 29. Pan-fried whole wheat spaghetti 30. Fresh nori nitsuke (similar) 14. Daikon nuka pickles 329. Amasake crescent cookies
28. Wakame, onion, cabbage, carrot miso soup 1b. Pressure-cooked brown rice 324. Bok choy, onion, carrot, sake-kasu nitsuke with chirimen iriko 189. Corn bread 15. Chinese cabbage nuka pickles	**Wednesday, December 19**	1b. Pressure-cooked brown rice 60. Vegetable oden 75. Northern white beans with miso 330. Takana pressed salad
28. Wakame, onion, carrot miso soup 1b. Pressure-cooked brown rice 155. Vegetable fritters (leftover) 13. Natto with pickled daikon leaves 14. Daikon nuka pickles	**Thursday, December 20**	1b. Pressure-cooked brown rice 323. Rice patties with miso 300. Green vegetable nitsuke 14. Daikon nuka pickles
18. Cauliflower leaves, onion, cabbage, carrot miso soup 1b. Pressure-cooked brown rice 140. Dried daikon nitsuke 330. Takana pressed salad	**Friday, December 21**	1b. Pressure-cooked brown rice 218. Cold salmon with gravy 80b. Clear soup with home-made tofu 21a. Tossed salad 330. Takana pressed salad
18. Turnip, onion, carrot miso soup 1b. Pressure-cooked brown rice 100. Okara nitsuke 300. Takana pressed salad	**Saturday, December 22**	1b. Pressure-cooked brown rice 29. Pan-fried noodles (leftover) 56. Garlic bread 140. Dried daikon nitsuke (leftover) 330. Takana pressed salad
Gone for entire day.	**Sunday, December 23**	*Gone for entire day.*

Breakfast		*Dinner*
18,29. Miso soup (leftover) *with* Fried noodles (leftover) 1b. Pressure-cooked brown rice 43. Burdock, lotus root, carrot kinpira 331. Toasted nori 15. Chinese cabbage nuka pickles	**Monday, December 24**	1b. Pressure-cooked brown rice 60. Vegetable oden (leftover) 75. Northern white beans (leftover) 21a. Tossed salad
Special Day - one meal only.	**Tuesday, December 25**	*Christmas Dinner* 41. Baked rice 167. Sesame spaghetti with oyster sauce 332. Pan-fried cod 114. Saifun salad 333. Tofu - egg clear soup 168. Baked potato with raw milk butter 81. White buns 334. Fruit cake
18. Daikon, onion, carrot miso soup 1b. Pressure-cooked brown rice 85. Chinese cabbage, wild spinach, onion, carrot nitsuke 14. Daikon nuka pickles	**Wednesday, December 26**	1b. Pressure-cooked brown rice 36. Casserole made from leftover cooked food 14,15. Daikon, cabbage nuka pickles
18. Daikon, onion, carrot miso soup 1b. Pressure-cooked brown rice 55. Cabbage nitsuke 14. Daikon, daikon leaves nuka pickles	**Thursday, December 27**	1b. Pressure-cooked brown rice 66,37. Boiled broccoli (similar) *with* Bechamel sauce 30. Nori nitsuke 15. Chinese cabbage nuka pickles 135. Amasake doughnuts
18. Daikon, onion, carrot miso soup 1b. Pressure-cooked brown rice 43. Vegetable kinpira (leftover) 13. Natto with pickled daikon leaves 15. Chinese cabbage nuka pickles	**Friday, December 28**	1b. Pressure-cooked brown rice 29. Pan-fried whole wheat spaghetti 21a. Tossed salad 14. Daikon nuka pickles 135. Amasake doughnuts 329. Amasake crescent cookies

Breakfast		Dinner
18. Cabbage, onion, carrot miso soup 1b. Pressure-cooked brown rice 54. Broccoli nitsuke 14. Daikon, daikon leaves nuka pickles	**Saturday, December 29**	1b. Pressure-cooked brown rice 53,22a. Udon *with* Tempura 48. Parsnip, celery nitsuke 14. Daikon nuka pickles 329. Apple butter crescent cookies (similar)
18. Cabbage, onion, carrot miso soup 1b. Pressure-cooked brown rice 22a. Tempura (leftover) 86. Fresh daikon nitsuke 15. Chinese cabbage nuka pickles	**Sunday, December 30**	1b. Pressure-cooked brown rice 29. Fried noodles (leftover) 133. Yam, carrot nitsuke 14. Daikon nuka pickles
18. Miso soup (leftover) 1b. Pressure-cooked brown rice 331. Toasted nori 85. Chinese cabbage nitsuke 14. Daikon, daikon leaves nuka pickles	**Monday, December 31**	1b. Pressure-cooked brown rice 50. Millet with chick pea sauce 72. Nori kombu nitsuke 15. Chinese cabbage nuka pickles

Glossary

Age: deep-fried tofu.

Amasake: a sweet drink made by fermenting cooked sweet rice with koji enzyme.

Azuki: small dark red bean grown mostly in Japan.

Bancha (twig) tea: tea made from the older leaves of the tea bush. Tea made from the younger leaves is *sencha.*

Burdock: long dark root vegetable, called *gobo* in Japanese.

Chirashi sushi: cooked rice with vegetables sprinkled on top. *Chirashi* means scatter.

Chirimen iriko: small dried fish used for soup stock.

Chuba iriko: small dried fish harvested in Chuba (now Iwate prefecture), Japan.

Daikon: large white Japanese radish.

Fuku musubi: stuffed and wrapped up, then tied with kampyo. *Fuku* means 'treasure.'

Fu: dried wheat gluten.

Goma ai: a cold cooked vegetable dish with sesame dressing. *Ai* means mixed and *goma* is sesame seed.

Gomashio: a condiment made from sesame seeds and salt. *Shio* is salt.

Gomoku rice: cooked rice combined with 5 or more ingredients. *Gomoku* means '5 kinds.'

Hijiki: dark bushy seaweed native of Japan belonging to the brown algae family.

Kampyo: edible dried gourd strips used for tying food.

Kanten: gelatin made from seaweed, called agar-agar in this country.

Karinto: a dessert or snack made by deep-frying rolled-out dough.

Kasha: buckwheat groats.

Kayu: grain cooked for a long time in a lot of water until soft and creamy.

Kinako: soybeans roasted and then ground.

Kinpira: a burdock dish.

Kinton: a dessert of mashed sweet potatoes or yams and whole chestnuts. It's like a pudding.

Kirigoma: roasted and cut (chopped) sesame seeds.

Koi-koku: a classic traditional stew made from fresh whole carp and burdock root. *Koi* is carp and *koku* means thick.

Kokkoh: grain cereal for babies (see *Macrobiotic Child Care).*

Kombu: seaweed of the brown algae family grown in long streamers which lay along the bottom in deep intertidal waters. *Dashi kombu* is a tough variety used to flavor soup stock. *Nishime kombu* is more tender and is used as a vegetable.

Konnyaku: a clear amber jelly-like cake made from konnyaku yam starch.

Kuzu: starch extracted from the root of a Japanese wild plant.

Matsuba: pine leaves.

Mekabu: root of wakame, rich in minerals.

Miso: soybeans, salt and a grain (rice, wheat, barley) which have been fermented together with a special enzyme.

Mochi: usually means steamed sweet rice which has been pounded and formed into balls or cakes. Mochi is traditionally served at New Year's.

Musubi: food which has been pressed or tied in some way.

Natto: fermented unsalted soybeans, popular for breakfast in Japan.

Nigari: liquid which drips from damp sea salt. High in magnesium chloride, used in the preparation of tofu. Available at natural food stores.

Nishime: style of cooked vegetables. They are cut in fairly large pieces, cooked slowly and seasoned with soy sauce.

Nitsuke: vegetables cut fairly small and cooked for a short time.

Nori: seaweed of red algae family. Delicate leafy, brownish plant grown in intertidal zones and cultivated in Japan.

Norimake sushi: rice rolled in nori.

Oden: traditional Japanese stew.

Ohagi: small balls of lightly pounded sweet rice often covered with sesame seeds or azuki beans or kinako. Traditionally served at spring and autumn equinox.

Ohitashi: lightly boiled vegetables.

Ojiya: rice porridge with vegetables — usually leftover rice and soup cooked together.

Okara: soybeans from which the milk has been extracted to make tofu.

Polenta: corn meal.

Saifun: clear noodles made from mung beans, often called bean threads or *harusame*. Orientals call them longevity noodles because they look like silver hair on an old person.

Sake: Japanese rice wine.

Sake-kasu: Paste left after making sake.

Sarashinegi: scallions chopped and passed under water.

Seitan: wheat gluten (fu) sauteed with tamari and ginger.

Shiro uri: Japanese cucumber with tender skin. *Uri* is cucumber, *shiro* is white.

Shiso: Japanese plant whose seeds and leaves are used for flavor.

Shiitake: type of large Japanese mushroom usually available in dried form.

Shingiku: garland chrysanthemum cultivated in the Orient for food. Available in Oriental food stores. If not available, watercress can be used.

Soba: buckwheat noodles.

Somen: Thin wheat summer noodles.

Sukiyaki: a style of noodle stew cooked at the table.

Suribachi: bowl with ridged inner surface used for grinding seeds and other foods.

Suricogi: wooden pestle used with suribachi.

Sushi: cooked rice flavored with rice vinegar, umeboshi or lemon juice – usually served cold for hot weather.

Takana: Japanese mustard green.

Takuan: daikon (dried outside) nuka pickle made in winter.

Tamari: traditional soy sauce *(shoyu)* made without chemicals.

Tazukuri: small dried blue fish.

Tekka: condiment of miso and vegetables cooked a long time.

Tempura: style of cooking whereby vegetables are dipped in batter and deep-fried.

Tofu: curdled soy milk.

Togan: Chinese cucumber squash.

Udon: large wheat flour noodles.

Uosuki: fish and vegetable stew cooked at the table.

Wakame: kelp-type seaweed of the brown algae family, native of Japan.

Yang: contracted by its nature or by 'yangization' — for example: time, pressure, salt or heat.

Yannoh: grain 'coffee' (see *Chico San Cookbook*).

Yin: expanded by its nature or by 'yinnization' — for example: raw, water, oil, or cold.

Index

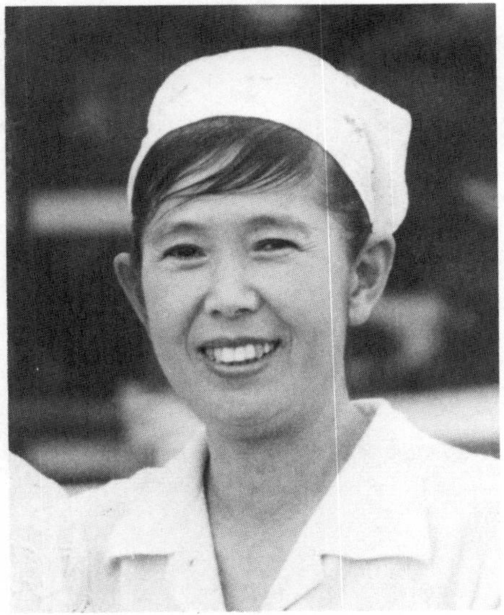

Cornellia Aihara learned the traditional arts of country-style food preparation at her native home in Aizuwakamatu (Fukushima prefecture), northern Japan. To this she added an understanding of healthful food combining and balancing according to yin and yang principles – an education she received later at the George Ohsawa macrobiotic school in Tokyo.

In 1955 she came to the United States and married Herman Aihara, founder of the George Ohsawa Macrobiotic Foundation. Their daughter Mari was born in 1958 and their son Jiro in 1959. At the first American macrobiotic summer camps in 1960, 61, 63, and 64 Cornellia studied cooking while assisting Mrs. Lima Ohsawa.

Since 1960 Cornellia has devoted her life to the teaching of macrobiotic cooking and philosophy. She has travelled extensively with her husband, giving cooking classes and lectures throughout the United States. She has become a foremost teacher of natural foods cooking and is well-known as a creator of balanced, healthful and delicious meals in harmony with nature.